Proceedings of the 20t

MW01595769

Functional and Chronic Diseases: Bioactive Compounds and Biomarkers

Organized by Functional Food Center

Functional and Medical Foods for Chronic Diseases: Bioactive Compounds and Biomarkers

Volume 20

Functional Food Center Inc./Functional Food Institute
7575 Frankford Rd, Dallas, TX 75252, USA
http://www.functionalfoodscenter.net

Printed and Edited in the United States of America

Copyright ©2016 by Food Science Publisher/ Danik M. Martirosyan

ISBN-13: 978-1537425528; ISBN-10: 1537425528

For information regarding special discounts for bulk purchases, please contact Food Science Publisher Special Sales at 469-441-8272 or email ffc@functionalfoodcenter.com

Important Notice:
This publication is neither a medical guide nor manual for self-treatment. If you should suspect that you suffer from a medical problem, you should seek competent medical care. The reader should consult his or her health professional before adopting any of the suggestions in this book.

Food Science Publisher 2016

Edited by Danik Martirosyan, PhD and Bruce Burnett, PhD

ACKNOWLEDGMENTS

I would like to extend our warmest gratitude to each contributor of this book for having shared his or her abstracts with us. We have included abstracts authored by esteemed experts from many different countries, including: Australia, Argentina, Bangladesh, Brazil, Colombia, Canada, China, Germany, Hong Kong, India, Italy, Iran, Japan, Lebanon, Mexico, Poland, Republic of Korea, Spain, Thailand, Turkey, UK, the USA and more.

It is our hope that those who read this book will become more knowledgeable about functional and medical foods, bioactive compounds, and biomarkers for the prevention, management, and treatment of chronic diseases.

Special thanks to the members of our organizing committee: Manoj K. Bhasin, PhD, Department of Medicine, Division of Interdisciplinary Medicine and Biotechnology, Beth Israel Deaconess Medical Center, Harvard Medical School, Boston, MA, USA; Francine Welty, MD, PhD, Associate Professor of Medicine at Harvard Medical School, Board-Certified Cardiologist at Beth Israel Deaconess Medical Center, Boston, MA, USA; Jin-Rong Zhou, PhD, Associate Professor of Surgery, Harvard Medical School, Director, Nutrition/Metabolism Laboratory, Beth Israel Deaconess Medical Center, Boston, MA, USA; John W. Froehlich, PhD, Harvard Medical School, Urology Department at Children's Hospital, Boston, MA, USA; Daniela Buscariollo, MD, Harvard Radiation Oncology Program, Harvard Radiation Oncology Social Committee Leader, Boston, MA, USA; Hoyoku Nishino, MD, PhD, Professor, Kyoto Prefectural University of Medicine, President, International Union of Wellness Science, President, Beautiful Life Science Society, Kyoto, Japan; Hiroshi Maeda, MD, PhD, Professor, Institute of Drug Delivery Science, Sojo University, Nishi-ku, Kumamoto, Japan; Nancy J. Emenaker, PhD, Program Director, Nutritional Science Research Group, Division of Cancer Prevention, National Cancer Institute, National Institutes of Health (NIH), Bethesda, MD, USA; Yasuhito Shirai, PhD,

Professor, Graduate School of Agricultural Science, Department of Agrobioscience, Kobe University, Kobe, Japan; Elizabeth Johnson, PhD, Associate Professor, Gerald J. and Dorothy R. Friedman School of Nutrition Science and Policy at Tafts University, Somerville, MA, USA; Zhongyi Li, PhD, Principal Research Scientist, CSIRO Plant Industry, Canberra, Australia; Francesco Marotta, MD, PhD, Professor, ReGenera Research Group for Aging Intervention, Milan, Italy; Montenapoleone Medical Center, Milano, Italy; Garth L. Nicolson, PhD, Professor, President, Chief Scientific Officer and Research Professor of Molecular Pathology, The Institute for Molecular Medicine, S. Laguna Beach, CA, USA. We would like to thank these people and institutions for their passion in spreading the word about this year's conference and helping us gather support in our efforts.

Also, I would like to thank Functional Food Center (USA), Technology Networks: The Online Scientific Community, and the Academic Society of Functional Foods and Bioactive Compounds (USA), for their help in promoting and sponsoring our conference this year.

Danik M. Martirosyan, PhD, President of Functional Food Center/ Functional Food Institute, Dallas, TX, USA

INTRODUCTION

The Functional Food Center has successfully held 20 International Conferences, including this one, since 2004. We take special interest in enabling the assimilation of scientific knowledge at our conferences under the series "Functional Foods for the Prevention and Management of Chronic Diseases." The 20th International Conference was held September 22nd through the 23rd, 2016, in the Joseph B. Martin Conference Center at Harvard Medical School, Boston, MA USA. This conference was titled "Functional and Medical Foods for Chronic Diseases: Bioactive Compounds and Biomarkers".

Main Conference Topics Include:

1. Functional Food Definition and the Status of Functional Foods in Japan, China, USA, and other Countries
2. Health Claims: Nutraceutical, Functional and Medical Food Regulations
3. Functional Foods and Obesity
4. Functional Foods and Diabetes
5. Functional Foods and Neurological Disorders
6. Functional Foods and Cardiovascular Disease (CVD)
7. Functional Foods and Cancer
8. Probiotics, Prebiotics, and Cancer
9. Prevention and Management of Dementia
10. The Effects of Nutrition and Functional Foods for Ageing and Health
11. Roles of Food Derived Nitrite/Nitrate from Cured Meat to Vegetables, to Hypertensions and/or Antioxidant Effect
12. Functional and Medical Foods with Bioactive Compounds: Prevention and Management of Noncommunicable Diseases
13. Current Research and Development of New Functional Food Products

Functional Food's research has allowed modern society to evade the side effects of modern pharmaceuticals and the problems associated with treating chronic diseases through surgical procedures. Presented in this book are scientists, food manufacturers, and healthcare professionals who are committed to functional food research that have brought together ideas and research to treat chronic illnesses and improve the quality of life through the utilization of functional foods with bioactive compounds.

This book presents the discovery, sources, potential health benefits, and safety aspects of bioactive compounds and functional foods for chronic diseases, in addition to, the scientific research and development of novel functional food products. This issue not only preserves the numerous scientific concepts and contributions made in the field of functional food, but also lays the foundation for a field of science that will undoubtedly logarithmically expand in the coming years, changing modern society's relationship with medicine.

Danik M. Martirosyan, PhD, President of Functional Food Center/ Functional Food Institute, Dallas, TX, USA

CONTENTS

PART FIVE
FUNCTIONAL FOODS AND NEUROLOGICAL DISORDERS   67

PART 1:

Functional Food Definition and the Status of Functional Foods in Japan, China, USA and other Countries

NUTRACEUTICAL REGULATIONS IN THE UNITED STATES WITH A SPECIAL EMPHASIS ON GRAS (GENERALLY RECOGNIZED AS SAFE) STATUS AND LABEL CLAIMS

Debasis Bagchi[1,2]

[1]Department of Pharmacological and Pharmaceutical Sciences, University of Houston College of Pharmacy, Houston, TX, USA; [2]Cepham Research Center, Piscataway, NJ, USA

Keywords: Regulations, DSHEA, GRAS, Label Claims

Background: Nutraceuticals and health foods are diligently regulated by the USFDA, DSHEA, FTC and allied regulatory authorities. According to the Centers for Disease Control and Prevention, about 50% of all US adults consume dietary supplements including vitamins, minerals, dietary supplements and nutraceuticals. The overall sales of dietary supplements surpassed $30 billion in 2011. To food scientists and marketers, functional foods or dietary supplements are health foods that contain certain health-promoting effects beyond traditional nutrients. However, according to FDA, terms like functional foods, nutraceuticals, herbal supplements or aquaceuticals have no meaning in regulation or the law, and in fact, are regarded as "fanciful".

Objective: This presentation will provide an outline how nutraceuticals and functional foods are being regulated in the United States and how the different regulatory authorities are involved. The nutrition labeling and education act (NLEA 1990), which permitted health claims for food, had long been resisted by the FDA. FDA does not permit disease claims; however, Congress passed FDAMA (FDA Modernization Act, 1997) to liberalize the interpretation that FDA had mandated for health claims, by allowing the claims to be based on "authoritative scientific statements based on research confirmation" of qualified scientific bodies much like judgements of safety could be made by expert panels for GRAS substances.

Approach: In December 1999, FDA made the pivotal decision that there must be significant scientific agreement about the substances/disease relationship rather than the actual claim being made. Although the guidance was subsequently withdrawn, it was supplanted by guidance issued in January of 2009, which refers to 21 CFR 101.14.

Results: Currently, five types of health-related statements or claims are allowed to some extent on functional food and dietary supplement labels including (i) nutrient content claims, (ii) structure and function claims, (iii) dietary guidance claims, (iv) qualified health claims, (v) health claims as approved by FDA and supported by significant scientific agreement. The salient features of insignificant agreement, emerging agreement, scientific agreement and general agreement (consensus) will be demonstrated with a special emphasis on DSHEA. Finally, the resolution to the impasse of the safety standard, type of claim, level of evidence for supporting efficacy, deciding body and recommendation for public disclosure will be discussed with respect to the health claims for functional foods and dietary supplements with selected examples.

Conclusion: Furthermore, a number of regulatory changes are being mandated in the United States at the end of 2015, which will unveil opportunities for novel well-researched nutraceuticals and dietary supplements.

FDA HEALTH CLAIMS FOR FOODS AND DIETARY SUPPLEMENTS

Paula Trumbo

PhD Nutrition Programs, US Food and Drug Administration

FDA does not have a definition for functional foods. But assuming that functional foods are foods that have a potentially positive effect on health beyond basic nutrition, then such foods, and the relevant components, are evaluated for health claims. Health claims are statements about the relationship between a food or food component and its role in disease risk, rather than about preventing a nutrient deficiency. Therefore, health claims can pertain to foods that contain nutrients that are not essential in the diet. For example, FDA has authorized several health claims for dietary fibers, as well as a health claim for phytosterols. In addition, FDA has issued qualified health claims for foods and nutrients (EPA/DHA) that are not essential in the diet.

CREATING NEW FUNCTIONAL FOOD PRODUCTS USING FFC'S NEW DEFINITION. RECENT DEVELOPMENTS ON NEW FORMULATIONS BASED ON OMEGA 3, VITAMIN C, AND SQUALENE

April Mitchell and Danik Martirosyan

Functional Food Institute, Dallas, TX, 75252, USA

Keywords: Functional food definition, Functional food products, Omega 3, Vitamin C, Squalene

The onset of the public and consumers becoming more health conscious and looking to new ways to become healthier, has spurred the rapidly growing field of functional food research for the prevention of chronic diseases and health promotion. Although the research and development of functional food products are being studied around the world, there is still not a globally accepted definition of functional food. Varying definitions in the literature and ambiguous government legislation have posed challenges for the development of functional food science and new effective functional food products for the consumer market. Here, the Functional Food Center defines "functional foods" as "Natural or processed foods that contains known or unknown biologically-active compounds; which, in defined, effective non-toxic amounts, provide a clinically proven and documented health benefit for the prevention, management, or treatment of chronic disease" [1,2]. This new definition of functional food by the Functional Food Center can improve the communication between the scientific and medical communities, food industry, and public. Thereby, improving the development of safe and effective new functional food products.

Since 1998, Functional Food Center has investigated and created innovative healthy food products and formulations. While working closely with UT Southwestern Medical Center and Texas Woman's University, over 70 formulations have successfully been tested for the efficacy of various bioactive compounds in mice models and clinical trials. From 1999 to 2010, FFC produced healthy products enriched with protein for athletes, dietary fibers and other bioactive compounds for the management of diabetes, and created gluten free products. These products include: quality muffin batter, pancake mixes, pizza dough, breads, and healthy drinks rich with probiotics, vitamin C, vitamin D, minerals such as iron, potassium, magnesium and bioactive compounds (Squalene, Lycopene, GOPO, and more).

Now, we are working on improving some of our health-related products and functional food formulations. One investigation involves Rose Hip (*Rosa canina L*) and its functional properties. Rose Hip is high in Vitamin C and also contains carotenoids, lycopene, tocopherol, bioflavonoids, tannins, pectin, sugars, organic acids, amino acids, and essential oils. Additionally, various studies have shown the beneficial effects of Rose Hip for Osteoarthritis (OA), Rheumatoid Arthritis (RA), and other chronic diseases [3]. Another healthy formulation includes Amaranth and the bioactive compound, Squalene, for the prevention of cardiovascular diseases [4].

References:

1. Martirosyan DM (Ed): Proceedings of the the 8th International Conference on Functional foods and Chronic Diseases: Science and Practice: March 15-17, 2011: Las Vegas, University of Nevada Las Vegas: Page 20
2. Danik M. Martirosyan and Jaishree Singh, A new definition of functional food by FFC: what makes a new definition unique? Functional Foods in Health and Disease 2015; 5(6):209-223
3. Cui Fan, Callen Pacier, Danik M. Martirosyan. Rose hip (Rosa canina L): A functional food perspective. Functional Foods in Health and Disease 2014; 4(11):493-509.
4. Martirosyan, D.M., Miroshnichenko, L.A., Kulakova, S.N., Pogojeva, A.V. and Zoloedov, V.I., 2007. Amaranth oil application for coronary heart disease and hypertension. *Lipids in health and disease*, 6(1), p.1.

Part 2
Health Claims: Nutraceutical, Functional and Medical Food Regulations

MEDICAL FOODS: AN ESSENTIAL THERAPEUTIC CATEGORY IN SEARCH OF DEFINITION AND FDA CLARIFICATION IN THE UNITED STATES

Bruce P. Burnett[1,2]

[1]The Nutrition and MF Coalition, Washington, D.C. 20002; USA;
[2]Entera Health, Inc., Cary, NC 27518, USA

Keywords: Distinctive Nutritional Requirement, Investigational New Drug, Generally Recognized as Safe (GRAS)

Medical foods (MFs) were first regulated as "dietary drugs", reviewed and approved for safety under the 1938 Federal Food, Drug, and Cosmetic Act (FFDCA). The first MF in name was Lofenalac®, a specially formulated meal replacement therapy with low phenylalanine approved by the FDA under FFDCA §201(g)(1)(B) in 1957 for management of phenylketonuria. All older MFs were approved under FFDCA §201(g)(1)(B) prior to modernization of the FDA in the 1960s requiring phase I-III trials. During the years of 1972-74, the FDA converted most MFs to "foods for special dietary use" (21 CFR 125, 1974; currently defined under 21 CFR 105, 2005). These are foods which do not require physician supervision, but provided needed nutrients for special situations to: (a) "supply a particular dietary requirement which exist by reason of a physical, physiological, pathological or other condition, including but not limited to the conditions of diseases, convalescence, pregnancy, lactation, allergic hypersensitivity to food, underweight, and overweight; (ii) Uses for supplying particular dietary needs which exist by reason of age, including but not limited to the ages of infancy and childhood; (iii) Uses for supplementing or fortifying the ordinary or usual diet with any vitamin, mineral, or other dietary property." Other MFs remaining in the drug category were generally recognized as safe

(GRAS), but subject to the same requirements as drugs. This led to a lack of development in this category of therapeutics.

Presumably in an effort to spur development of MFs, an amendment was added to the 1988 update to the Orphan Drug Act (21 U.S.C. 360ee(b)(3)), which established the MF category separate from FDA-approved drugs and Foods for Special Dietary Use. Creation of the MF category occurred six years in advance of the establishment of the dietary supplement category in 1994 under the Dietary Supplement Health and Education Act (21 U.S.C. § 301). The Orphan Drug Act defined MFs as "a food which is formulated to be consumed or administered enterally under the supervision of a physician and which is intended for the specific dietary management of a disease or condition for which distinctive nutritional requirements, based on recognized scientific principles, are established by medical evaluation." In 1991, the MF category was reaffirmed in the Nutrition Labeling and Education Act (NLEA; see 21 U.S.C. 343 (q) (5) (A) (iv)) which further defined the MFs, but exempted these products from the nutrition labeling required for conventional foods. The NLEA was also the basis for the regulation which the FDA developed for MFs stated in 21 CFR 101.9 (j)(8) finalized in 1993. This regulation further defined the category requiring that a food is a MF exempt from nutrition labeling only if:

a) "It is a specially formulated and processed product (as opposed to a naturally occurring foodstuff used in its natural state) for the partial or exclusive feeding of a patient by means of oral intake or enteral feeding by tube;

b) It is intended for the dietary management of a patient who, because of therapeutic or chronic medical needs, has limited or impaired capacity to ingest, digest, absorb, or metabolize ordinary foodstuffs or certain nutrients, or who has other special medically determined nutrient requirements, the dietary management of which cannot be achieved by the modification of the normal diet alone;

c) It provides nutritional support specifically modified for the management of the unique nutrient needs that result from the specific disease or condition, as determined by medical evaluation;

d) It is intended to be used under medical supervision; and

e) It is intended only for a patient receiving active and ongoing medical supervision wherein the patient requires medical care on a recurring basis for, among other things, instructions on the use of the MF."

In 1996, the FDA issued proposed regulations meant to define certain terms in the Orphan

Drug Act, the NLEA and from 21 CFR 101.8(j)(8). The Advance Notice of Proposed Rulemaking (ANPR; FDA-CFSAN Federal Register 61 FR 60661, November 29, 1996) contained suggested definitions for a "distinctive nutritional requirement," language on what constituted evidence of efficacy and "medical supervision" for MFs and was discussed publically for seven years until 2003 when it was withdrawn by the FDA without further action. This was the last time that the FDA proposed real regulation for MFs. In 2007, the FDA issued nonbinding guidance in the form of Frequently Asked Questions (FAQs) in attempt to advise industry and others on what constituted MFs, but this document did nothing to define terms in the Orphan Drug Act of 1988, the NLEA and from 21 CFR 101.8(j)(8) or to provide guidance on what constitutes proof for a "distinctive nutritional requirement" or clinical trial evidence. In 2008, the FDA finalized a MF Program Guidance Manual to be used by its field inspectors in case they encountered MF products at drug production facilities. This manual restated the content of the previous laws and guidance documents, prevented the import of MFs from overseas, gave the drug inspectors guidance on how to sample products and inspect labels. In 2013, the FDA further suggested in an update to the FAQs that MFs were appropriate for inborn errors of metabolism, but not for diabetics or pregnancy. The guidance also stated that MFs could not be Rx only, a drug distinction. It restated that MFs required medical or physician supevision. This guidance was finalized in May 2016. The drug division at FDA in 2013 also issued guidance to institutional review boards which required the industry to obtain an investigational new drug application (IND) to perform a clinical study.

The FAQ guidance on MFs provided no direction for the marketing or definition for MFs. In addition, the FAQ guidance has also created confusion for drug listing agencies now requiring MFs to become OTC products, payers who are dropping coverage and physicians, pharmacists as well as patients who have had their access to MFs limited by FDA inaction. Further, the IND guidance requiring medical foods to file a drug application has prevented manufacturers from executing clinical trials to substantiate claims to avoid action by the Federal Trade Commission as a MF. Industry has formed a Nutrition and Medical Food Coalition to propose "best practices" in the development and marketing of MFs toward an eventual FDA-approval process in the future.

HEALTH CLAIMS ON FOOD PACKAGING – LITTLE APPARENT NEED FROM SOUTH AUSTRALIAN ADULTS

Malcolm Riley [1], Jane Bowen [1], Debra Krause [2], Darren Jones [3] and Welma Stonehouse [1]

[1]Food and Nutrition, Commonwealth Scientific and Industrial Research Organisation, South Australian Health and Medical Research Institute, Adelaide, 5000, Australia; [2]Food and Nutrition, Commonwealth Scientific and Industrial Research Organisation, Sneydes Rd, Werribee, Victoria, 3030, Australia; [3]Information Management & Technology, Commonwealth Scientific and Industrial Research Organisation, Waite Campus, Urrbrae, 5001, Australia;

Keywords: health claims, adults, South Australia, food packaging

Background: Australia has for many decades required a Nutrient Information Panel to be included on food packaging, usually on the back. Recently, a health rating system has been developed for use on food packaging, and a regulated system for making health claims about the food on packaging has been legislated. The scope for these new initiatives to acheive their purpose depends on how they are percieved and trusted by consumers. This report describes the results of a population based survey of South Australian adults about how the food label is used to inform purchase decisions.

Objective: To understand the attitudes and views of South Australian adults to information provided on food packaging.

Methods: A survey was conducted using a random stratified sampling technique in people aged 15 years and older in the Australian state of South Australia. All surveys were administered face-to-face to 3005 people between September 2015 and December 2015. Data were weighted by the inverse of the individual's probability of selection, as well as the response rate in metropolitan and country regions and then reweighted to benchmarks from the June 2014 Estimated Resident Population calculated by the Australian Bureau of Statistics.

Results: The response rate for the survey was 57.3%. Most respondents to the survey rated their own dietary intake as 'healthy' (61.5%) or 'extremely healthy' (9.1%). Country of origin was nominated as the most important information looked for on the food label of a food bought for the first time (by 35%), followed by the ingredient list (21.6%) and claims about nutrition (20.9%). The response to this question was markedly different by age group, with almost half (48.3%) of those aged 55 years or over considering that country of origin was the most important information to look for. For the youngest age group (15-34 yrs) 28.4% considered the ingredient list was the most important information, 26.5% considered claims about nutrition to be most important and only 22.2% considered country of origin to be the most important information on the food label. The Nutrition Information Panel was used to guide purchase decision for a new breakfast cereal by more than half of respondents (50.8%). 44.0% disagreed (36.1% disagreed somewhat, 17.9% disagreed completely) that 'statements about health on food packaging are a trustworthy source of information', however only 22.1% disagreed (16.4% disagreed somewhat, 5.7% disagreed completely) with the statement that 'the Nutrient Information Panel on food packaging is a trustworthy source of information'.

Conclusion: For South Australian adults, statements about health benefits of food on food packaging are viewed with greater suspicion than statements about the nutrient content of food. Views on food packaging varied more by age group than by sex of the respondent. For an unfamiliar food, country of origin is considered the most important information on food packaging by more than a third of adults.

NUTRACEUTICAL REGULATIONS IN THE SOUTHEAST ASIAN SUBCONTINENT

Narendra Deshmukh

INTOX Pvt. Ltd., Pune, India

Keywords: Nutraceutical regulations, Southeast Asia (SEA), nutritional deficiency, Codex Alimentarius guidelines

The region of Southeast Asia (SEA), home to 625 million people, is replete with natural resources, geographical and ethnic diversity and a long history, in which are rooted its rich and healthy food traditions. Especially, SEA is a pioneer in recognizing foods with potential health benefits for centuries, which is now known as nutraceuticals and functional foods. The region shares a number of naturally grown foods eaten traditionally across SEA countries and India, the land where "Ayurveda" was conceptualized. The philosophy of Ayurveda teaches a series of conceptual systems characterized by balance and disorder, health and disease.

Closely following regulations on Traditional Medicines, the Food Regulations in the region have evolved while responding to a diversity of factors. For instance, malnutrition caused by socio-economic disparities and by endemic nutritional deficiencies, prompted regulations on food fortification and nutrition labeling. While regulations were also made for religious reasons like Islamic purity law-Halal, most have been made to protect the consumers.

There are variations in food and nutraceutical regulations across the region, though in most countries these were developed following Codex Alimentarius guidelines. In more recent times, with improved socio-economic conditions, new regulations are prompted by entry of processed foods with various functional claims and risk avoidance benefits. Some of these are similar to those in more regulated markets such as Europe, US or Canada. In general, though functional foods are yet not well defined and regulated in many of the countries, the regulations are now seen being revised in response to the emerging concerns for safety, efficacy and quality.

Overall, nutrient must be present in Health Foods and Nutraceuticals in certain quantities. Health claims are not permitted under current food regulations. However, the authorities are examining the Codex document on health claims and developing claims that can be used in support of structurally diverse nutraceuticals and functional foods.

Part 3
Functional Foods and Obesity

CLINICAL EFFICACY OF A NOVEL GREEN COFFEE BEAN EXTRACT (GCB-70) IN OVERWEIGHT SUBJECTS

Manashi Bagchi[1], Narsingh Verma[2], Madhukar Mittal[3], Anand Swaroop[1], Debasis Bagchi[1,4], Pawan Kumar[5] and Harry G. Preuss[6]

[1]Cepham Research Center, Piscataway, NJ, USA; [2]Department of Physiology, KG Medical University, Lucknow, UP, India; [3]Department of Medicine, KG Medical University, Lucknow, UP, India; [4]University of Houston College of Pharmacy, Houston, TX, USA; [5]Chemical Resources, Panchkula, Haryana, India; [6]Georgetown University Medical Center, Washington, DC, USA.

Keywords: GCB-70, t-chlorogenic acid (CGA), caffeoylquinic acid, body weight, BMI (body mass index), waist circumference (WC), HbA1c, plasma leptin, safety

Background: Overweight and obesity is now a worldwide epidemic and a novel natural therapeutic intervention is warranted. We have developed a novel, patent-pending (PCT/IN2015/000236 dated 10th June 2015), water-soluble green coffee bean extract, GCB-70) enriched in 70% total chlorogenic acid including 45% caffeoylquinic acid and <1% caffeine in our laboratories. Our earlier studies demonstrated its novel antioxidant efficacy and its potential efficacy in weight management in rodents. This open-labelled investigation evaluated the efficacy of GCB-70 in 100 men and women overweight subjects (age: 18-65 years; body weight: 84.04 ± 1.46 kg) and BMI; 31.45 ± 4.49 kg/m^2) over a period of 12 weeks.

Methods: Institutional Review Board (IRB) and other institutional regulatory approvals were obtained for this study. This study was also registered in www.clinicaltrials.gov NCT02703025   Unique

Protocol ID: Protocol #CR-GCB- 70/ 07/14). Capsules (500 mg each, b.d.) were administered by the subjects 30-60 min prior to lunch and dinner. This study examined the body weight, BMI, WC and fasting glucose at 0, 4, 8 and 12 weeks of treatment. HbA1c, plasma leptin levels and thyroid stimulating hormone (TSH) were assessed at 0 and 12 weeks of treatment. Furthermore, extensive blood chemistry, adverse events, and physical health of the subjects were extensively evaluated to demonstrate the broad spectrum safety of GCB-70.

Results: Body weight was reduced by 1.9%, 3.9% and 5.9% in male volunteers at 4, 8 and 12 weeks of treatment, respectively, while under these same conditions approximately 2.3%, 3.8% and 6.0% reductions were observed in female volunteers. BMI was reduced by 1.3%, 3.9% and 5.9% in male volunteers at 4, 8 and 12 weeks of treatment, respectively, while under these same conditions approximately 2.3%, 3.9% and 6.1% reductions were observed in female volunteers.

Significant reductions in WC and fasting glucose were observed at these same time points in both male and female volunteers. HbA1c and plasma leptin levels were significantly reduced at 90-days of treatments as compared to the corresponding baseline values, respectively. No adverse events were observed. Also, blood chemistry data demonstrated the broad spectrum safety of GCB-70

Conclusions: Overall, the results demonstrate that GCB-70 is novel, safe and low caffeine antioxidant supplement effective in healthy weight management.

POLYMANNURONIC ACID OF BROWN SEAWEED PREVENT OBESITY IN HIGH-FAT DIET MICE DUE TO ITS EFFECTS ON GUT MICROBIOTA

Qingjuan Tang, Fang Liu, and Changhu Xue

College of Food Science and Engineering, Ocean University of China, Qingdao, China, 266003, China

Keywords: Polymannuronic acid, Obesity, Gut microbiota, Inflammation

Background: Obesity, an important risk factor of inflammation and clinically diseases, is prevalent in different age groups. Chronic inflammation is considered as one of the primary mechanisms underlying obesity. Accumulating evidences suggest that gut microflora play a key role in the development of chronic inflammation and obesity. Recently, polysaccharides were reported to have the effects of restoring the disordered gut microbiota and thus prevent chronic inflammation and obesity. Polymannuronic acid (PM), $1 \to 4$ linked β-d-mannuronic acid, is a fraction of algae polysaccharides and has been widely used according to its variety of bioactivities. However, little is known about the effect of PM on obesity.

Objective: To clarify the effects of PM on obesity and understand the underlying mechanisms.

Methods: Male C57BL/6J mice were randomly distributed into four groups. Normal group (N): fed with a standard chow diet for 90 days. High-fat group (M): fed with high-fat diet for 60 days. High-fat + fructo-oligosaccharide group (FOS): fed with high-fat diet in the first 60 days, while in the last 30 days, the mice were given 150mg/kg fructo-oligosaccharide by gavage once a day with high-fat diet simultaneously. High-fat + polymannuronic acid

(PM): fed with high-fat diet in the first 60 days, while in the last 30 days, the mice were given 150mg/kg PM by gavage once a day with high-fat diet simultaneously. Serum blood triglyceride and glucose were measured with specific reagent kits. Serum LPS levels were measured by ELISA method. Genes associated with inflammation, including IL-10, TNF-α, CD-11c, and MCP-1, were detected by Real-Time quantitative PCR. The change of gut microbiota induced by PM was detected by high-throughput sequencing and analyzed by bioinformatics. Short-chain fatty acids were detected by gas chromatography.

Results: The results showed that PM resisted the development of chronic inflammation and obesity induced by high-fat diet in C57BL/6J mice. PM treatment reduced blood triglyceride levels and improved glucose tolerance in HFD-fed mice. Endotoxins were significantly retarded after administrated with PM. The inflammation in colon and eAT was also alleviated. The diversity of gut microbiota in PM-treated mice was changed significantly. Anti-inflammatory microbiota -Lactobacillus, Ruminococcaceae, Bifidobacteriaceae and Akkermansia.muciniphila were increased and pro-inflammatory microbiota Proteobacteria was decreased. Butyrate, which has the effect of anti-inflammatory gut bacteria metabolites, as well as butyrate-producing bacteria - Eubacterium and Ruminococcus were increased after PM treatment.

Conclusion: PM has positive effects on preventing high-fat diet induced chronic inflammation and obesity. These effects may be attributed to its regulation of chronic inflammation mediated by intestinal flora. Our study revealed that PM might serve as a new prebiotics to reconstruct the disordered gut microbiota.

EFFECT OF DIFFERENT CONCENTRATIONS OF PROTEINS IN A SOLUBLE HIGH FIBER FOOD ON THE SHORT-TERM SATIETY IN HEALTHY YOUNG ADULTS

Palma XE[1], Oliveri MA[1], Araya H[1]

[1]Universidad de Valparaíso, Facultad de Farmacia, Escuela de Nutrición y Dietética Av. Gran Bretaña 1093, Valparaíso, Playa Ancha

Keywords: Soluble fiber, proteins, satiety, energy intake

Background: In response to a meal composition, the body releases different hormones that signal the hypothalamus to contribute to the cessation of eating. Satiety is defined as the state of eating cessation and it is associated with a delay in the initiation of subsequent meal so it has a direct effect on food and energy intake. There is general consensus that meals higher in protein produce greater satiety than meals high in either carbohydrates or fats. Proposed mechanisms include mechanical distention of the stomach, incretin responses from the small intestine, neurotransmitter responses in the brain, fuel changes in the hypothalamus, and leptin production. Amino acid sensing is believed to contribute to the homeostatic regulation of food intake and body weight. On the other hand, dietary fibers, including soluble and insoluble, benefit human health through their effects on satiety, glycemia, gut microflora composition, and lipid profile. The mechanism of action of soluble fiber intake on lower body weight is related to its effect on FI by forming gels in the gastrointestinal tract, thereby delaying digestion and absorption of other macronutrients and through gastric distension.

Objective: To test if an increase in protein content of a food rich in soluble fiber can improve satiety, we analyze the effect of 3 different concentrations of calcium caseinate on a flaxseed based muffin over short-term satiety in young adults.

Methods: A randomized 3-condition study was conducted in 22 healthy young men (mean age: $22 \pm 2{,}6$ y). Isocaloric muffins were prepared with the same amount of a mixture 1:1 of whole flaxseed flour (high in soluble fiber) and refined wheat flour and 3 different concentrations of calcium caseinate: 0% (control), 8% (C1) y 14% (C2). Each session, subjects arrived at the laboratory 3 hours after having a standard breakfast and ate one cf the three muffins. One hour later, subjects were offered an ad libitum hot lunch meal (spaghetti and meat sauce) and were instructed to eat as much as they wanted to feel comfortably satiated. 10-cm visual analogue scales (VAS scores) were used to assess hunger, satiety, fullness, prospective food consumption, and desires for something salty, sweet, or fatty after the consumption of the test muffin and before and after lunch. Objective food intake was measured by differential weighting between the amount of food served and left over in each plate.

Results were statistically analyzed by repeated measures ANOVA, T-paired (parametric) and Kruskal Wallis, Wilcoxon test (nonparametric).

Results: For the subjective evaluation, perception of hunger obtained after consumption of C2 was significantly lower compared to C ($p = 0{,}017$) and to C1 ($p = 0{,}013$). Something similar occurred when hunger was assessed before but not after lunch (data not shown). Accordingly, satiety and fullness were significantly higher after ingestion of C2 compared to C ($p = 0{,}032$ and $p < 0{,}01$, respectively) and before lunch ($p = 0{,}04$ and $p < 0{,}01$, respectively). There were no differences between C y C1. Desire to eat something and to eat something sweet showed a significant higher score after ingestion of control muffin compared with the 2 calcium caseinate added muffins. Food and energy intake were significantly lower after consumption of C2 muffins in relation to the other two.

Conclusion: Our study demonstrated that protein addition in a soluble fiber rich food increases satiety and fullness and decreases food and energy intake in young men. These results are important in showing an alternative to formulate healthy snacks that could be helpful in fighting obesity especially in children.

Part 4
Functional Foods and Diabetes

SAFETY AND EFFICACY OF A NOVEL FENUGREEK SEED (*TRIGONELLA FOENUM-GRAECUM,* FENFURO[TM]) EXTRACT IN PATIENTS WITH TYPE-2 DIABETES

Anand Swaroop[1], Manashi Bagchi[1], Pawan Kumar[2], Harry G. Preuss[3] and Debasis Bagchi[1,4]

[1]Cepham Research Center, Piscataway, NJ, USA; [2]Research & Development, Chemical Resources, Panchkula, Haryana, India; [3]Georgetown University Medical Center, Washington, DC, USA; [4]University of Houston College of Pharmacy, Houston, TX, USA

Keywords: Fenugreek, type 2 diabetes, clinical study, HbA1c, C-peptide levels

Background: *Trigonella foenum-graecum* seeds are known to exhibit potent antioxidant, hypoglycemic and nephroprotective activities, as well as serve as an excellent membrane stabilizer especially because of their content of novel furostanolic saponins. Our previous studies exhibited the broad spectrum safety and efficacy of Fenfuro, a novel *Trigonella foenum-graecum* seed extract enriched in furostanolic saponins, in type 2 diabetes (T2D) in rats.

Methods: This multi-center, randomized, placebo-controlled, double-blind, add-on clinical study evaluated over a period of 3 months the efficacy of Fenfuro (500 mg bid) in 154 male and female subjects (25-60 years) with T2D. This study examined the body weight, blood pressure and pulse rate, as well as the efficacy of Fenfuro on fasting and post-prandial plasma sugar, HbA1c and fasting and post-prandial C-peptide levels.

Results: Fenfuro caused significant reduction in both fasting plasma and post-prandial blood sugar levels. Approximately 83%

of the subjects reported decrease in fasting plasma sugar levels in the Fenfuro group as compared to 62% in the placebo group, while 89% of the subjects demonstrated reduction in post-prandial plasma sugar levels in the Fenfuro-treated group as compared to 72% in the placebo group. HbA1c levels were reduced in both placebo and treatment groups. The decrease in HbA1c levels was significant in both groups as compared to respective baseline values. A significant increase in fasting and post-prandial C-peptide levels compared to the respective baseline values, were observed, while no significant changes in fasting and post-prandial C-peptide levels were observed between the two groups. Extensive blood chemistry analyses exhibited the broad spectrum safety of Fenfuro. Furthermore, 48.8% subjects reported reduced dosage of anti-diabetic therapy in Fenfuro-treated group, while 18.05% reported reduced dosage of anti-diabetic therapy in the placebo-group.

Conclusion: In summary, Fenfuro proved safe and efficacious in ameliorating the symptoms of T2D in humans.

ORAL ADMINISTRATION OF EPIGALLOCATECHIN GALLATE (EGCG) IMPROVED DIABETIC NEPHROPATHY IN MICE

Daiki Hayashi, Shuji Ueda, Minoru Yamanoue, Hitoshi Ashida, and Yasuhito Shirai

Department of Applied Chemistry in Bioscience, Graduate School of Agricultural Science, Faculty of Agriculture, Kobe University, Japan

Keywords: catechins, diacylglycerol kinase, diabetic nephropathy

Background: Diabetic nephropathy is one of the diabetic vascular complications. It is known that diabetic vascular complications are caused by abnormal protein kinase C (PKC) activation delivered from diacylglycerol (DG), which is increased in diabetic hyperglycemia. On one hand, diacylglycerol kinase (DGK) converts DG to phosphatidic acid (PA). Therefore, activation of DGK may prevent and/or improve diabetic vascular complications. Actually, it was reported that vitamin E (VtE) improved diabetic nephropathy, by normalizing DG level and PKC activity through DGK activation. We revealed that, among the mammalian DGKs, DGK alpha (DGKα) was involved in the improvement of diabetic nephropathy by intraperitoneally administration of VtE in mice. Recently, we reported that galloylated catechins including epigallocatechin gallate (EGCg) also activated DGKα through 67 kDa laminin receptor (67LR) that is known as EGCg receptor (D. Hayashi, et al, Journal of Functional Foods, 2015, 15; 561-569). However, the effect of oral administration of EGCg on diabetic nephropathy remains unclear. Here, we examined whether oral administration of EGCg could improve diabetic nephropathy in diabetic mice.

Objective: To evaluate the effect of oral administration of EGCg on diabetic nephropathy, we fed EGCg-containing food to diabetic mice.

Methods: Six weeks old male wild type (WT) mice were divided into four groups as follows. Control group: non diabetic and normal food, Control+EGCg group: non diabetic and (1%) EGCg-containing food, STZ group: diabetic mice, that was intraperitoneal administered streptozotocin (STZ) and normal food, STZ+EGCg group: diabetic mice and (1%) EGCg food. To evaluate symptoms of diabetic nephropathy, we measured urine volume and urine albumin every week after the administering STZ or vehicle until 6 weeks. At the end of the experiment, mice were sacrificed and we measured kidney weight.

Results: First, we fed 1% EGCg-containing food to diabetic mice. There were no differences in blood glucose level between STZ group and STZ+EGCg group, indicating that EGCg did not improve diabetes itself. In diabetic nephropathy patients, it is well known that urine volume, urine albumin amount and kidney weight increase. In STZ group, urine volume, urine albumin amount and kidney weight increased by STZ treatment, but in the case of STZ+EGCg group, the symptoms were improved. Next, we tested lower concentration of EGCg. Then, we checked whether 0.05, 0.1, 0.5 % EGCg food improve diabetic nephropathy. As a result, at least 0.05 % EGCg (approximately 75 mg/kg body weight) food group showed significant decrease of urine volume and showed tendency to improve albuminuria.

Conclusion: In this study, we revealed that oral administration of EGCg could improve diabetic nephropathy. Moreover, the fact that oral administration of 0.05 % EGCg improved diabetic nephropathy in mice suggested that EGCg tablet might be functional food for diabetic nephropathy. Additionally, we reported that both of DGKα and 67LR are expressed in glomerular vascular epithelial cell (podocyte). Therefore, we evaluated the mechanisms of EGCg-induced improvement of diabetic nephropathy in podocyte.

COMPARING THE EFFECT OF MEMANTINE ON METABOLISM, OXIDATIVE STRESS AND ANTIOXIDANT RESERVES IN PATIENTS WITH MILD COGNITIVE IMPAIRMENT, WITH AND WITHOUT TYPE 2 DIABETES; AN EXPERIMENTAL CLINICAL TRIAL

Mehrdad Larry [1], Hossein Mirmiranpour[1], Alireza Esteghamati[1] and Manouchehr Nakhjavani[1]

[1]Endocrinology and Metabolism Research Center (EMRC), Imam Khomeini Hospital, Tehran University of Medical Sciences, Tehran, Iran

Keywords: memantine, oxidative stress, Alzheimer's disease, type 2 diabetes, clinical trial

Background: Connections between metabolic and oxidative mechanisms of Alzheimer's disease and diabetes have been previously demonstrated. Memantine blocks the N-methyl-d-aspartate (NMDA) receptor channels and has been clinically useful in Alzheimer's disease. It has also been determined to reduce oxidative stress as a non-competitive NMDA-receptor blocker. Treatment with memantine caused less microvascular changes in diabetic rats.

Objective: To determine if memantine has different affects on metabolic, oxidative and antioxidative properties of patients in early stages of Alzheimer's disease defined as mild cognitive impairment (MCI) versus patients with both MCI and type 2 diabetes.

Methods: The study consisted of three separate groups; healthy controls (C), patients with MCI and without diabetes (MCI), patients with MCI and type 2 diabetes (MCIT2D). Each group had 25 patients. The second and third groups were treated with memantine hydrochloride (up to 10 mg per day). Patients were followed for 6 months. Body mass index (BMI), waist circumference (WC), fasting blood glucose (FBS), hemoglobin A1c (HbA1c), systolic blood pressure (SBP), diastolic blood pressure (DBP), AGE (advanced glycation end products), AOPP (advanced oxidation protein products), FRAP (ferritin reducing ability of plasma), paraoxonase (PON), lipoprotein lipase (LPL), lecithin cholesterol acyltransferase (LCAT) were all measured before and after the follow-up. Pre-drug and post-drug characteristics and markers of oxidative stress for each group were compared by independent sample T-tests.

Results: Group MCI had higher SBP and lower levels of PON, LPL and LCAT compared with group C while group MCIT2D had lower levels of AGE and FRAP compared with group C. Group MCIT2D had higher HbA1c and SBP, but lower PON, LPL and LCAT activity compared with Group MCI at baseline. After follow-up, HbA1c decreased in both groups; FBS significantly reduced in MCIT2M group but did not change in MCI group (p-value<0.001 compared with 0.11, respectively). In both groups, SBP decreased significantly but DBP decreased in the MCIT2D group (p-value=0.02) and not in the MCI group (p-value=0.32). Serum levels of AOPP and FRAP did not change after treatment in any group. In group MCI, serum levels of AGE increased after the treatment while no significant change was observed in group MCIT2M. Activities of PON, LPL and LCAT were all increased after the treatment (p-values: 0.002, <0.001, <0.001 respectively) in group ADT2M. However, in group MCI, only LCAT had significantly increased (p-value= 0.04) and activities of both PON and LPL did not change.

Conclusion: MCI is partly due to oxidative stress and NMDA receptor overactivation. Similarly, in type 2 diabetes, hyperglycemic states and oxidative stress are the main causes of vascular complications. Memantine is more effective in the prevention of both metabolic and oxidative damage in patients who have type 2 diabetes as well as MCI.

SINGLE CHAIN ANTIBODIES AGAINST ADVANCED GLYCATION ENDPRODUCTS EVALUATED WITH SYNTHETICALLY MODIFIED PEPTIDES AND PROTEINS

Ulrika Wendel[1], Lena Danielsson[2], Nina Persson[1], Christian Risinger[1], Charlotte Welinder[3,4], Bo Jansson[3], Ola Blixt[1]

[1]Department of Chemistry, Faculty of Science, Copenhagen University, Denmark; [2]Clinical Chemistry and Pharmacology, Dept. of Laboratory Medicine, Lund University, Sweden; [3]Oncology and Pathology, Dept. of Clinical Sciences, Lund University, Lund, Sweden; [4]Centre of Excellence in Biological and Medical Mass Spectrometry "CEBMMS", Biomedical Centre D13, Lund University, Lund, Sweden.

Keywords: advanced glycation endproducts (AGE), chronic disease, peptide array, phage display, scFv, carbohydrates, Maillard reactions, diet, monoclonal antibodies.

Background: Advanced glycation endproducts (AGEs) are formed by spontaneous reactions between reactive sugars and protein-bound amino groups, typically found on lysine and arginine. The irreversible complex is a result of a series of chemical reactions known as the Maillard reactions (1). Formation of AGE-modified proteins is a frequent phenomenon in humans, known to induce oxidative stress and to trigger inflammatory response, by antibody production and binding to receptors (2). The consequences of advanced glycation are associated with chronic disease such as atherosclerosis, rheumatoid arthritis, diabetes, and cancer (3, 4). AGE structures are also commonly formed in processed foods containing carbohydrates and protein/fat, especially during heating (5). The glycation endproducts are then easily absorbed during the digestion of food, making an interesting connection between diet and chronic disease.

A limited number of monoclonal antibodies against different AGE modifications exist and there is an unmet need for a new generation of epitope-mapped antibodies to fill the specificity gap for improved analytical capacity and better diagnostics and therapeutics.

Objective: To develop highly specific scFv (single chain variable fragments) antibodies, which bind to AGE structures, using phage display. The binding-patterns of the scFv were evaluated with a large glycated peptide and protein microarray library and were then further validated on relevant biological material.

Methods: Phage display libraries (6, 7, 8) were obtained from mouse immunized with AGE-modified proteins (IgG and BSA modified with glucose, glyceraldehyde, methylglyoxal, glyoxal, glyoxylic acid and pyruvic acid). With a newly developed microarray selection and screening method (9) we obtained anti-AGE monoclonal antibodies that were further characterized using (i) comprehensive AGE-peptide and -protein microarrays and (ii) relevant cell lines and tissue microarrays.

Results: An immune response against AGE-structures was obtained in the serum of the immunized mouse. A larger AGE antigen library was used for the selection of phage displayed AGE antibodies. After conversion to soluble scFv, 600 of the selected antibodies were screened on a comprehensive array against the AGE modifications carboxymethyl lysine (CML) and carboxyethyl lysine (CEL). Twenty binding clones were further evaluated on a larger antigen array, containing the same antigens as in the phage selection. The binding patterns of these differed from the patterns of commercial CML- and CEL- antibodies.

Conclusion: New scFv antibodies against AGE-structures were generated and then evaluated by a microarray assay. Thereby obtained antibodies showed a difference in binding patterns compared to commercial antibodies. Well-defined and epitope-mapped antibodies against AGE are crucial for the development of new diagnostics and therapeutics and in the continuing investigation of glycation mechanism.

Funding: This work was supported by the Danish Research Council: DFF-4005-00285, the European Union, Seventh Framework Programme, GastricGlycoExplorer (GGE) initial training network: grant number 316929; and Innovationsfonden in the framework of the EU-ERASynBio project SynGlycTis; EbolaMoDRAD from Innovative Medicines Initiative (IMI2) No: 115843.

References:

1. Thornalley et.al., Biochemical Journal, no. 344(1999): 109–116.
2. Takahashi et.al, The Journal of Pharmacology and Experimental Therapeutics, no. 330(2009): 89–98.
3. Goldin et.al., Circulation, no. 114(2006): 597-605.
4. Sasaki et.al., The American Journal of Pathology, no.153(1998): 1149-55.
5. Liang et.al., Molecules, no. 463(2016).
6. Krebber et.al., Journal of Immunological Methods, no. 201(1997): 35-55.
7. Lindner and Plückthun, Antibody Engineering, Kontermann and Dübel, Eds., Springer-Verlag, Berlin Heidelberg (2001): 637-647.

8. Schaefer, Honegger, and Plückthun, Antibody Engineering, Kontermann and Dübel, Eds. Springer-Verlag, Berlin Heidelberg (2010): 21-44.

ISOTHIOCYANATES FROM THE EDIBLE PLANT NASTURTIUM AND THE PREVENTION OF TYPE 2 DIABETES: REDUCTION IN GLUCOSE PRODUCTION AND MODULATION OF PROTECTIVE PATHWAYS

Valentina Guzmán-Pérez[1,2], Christiane Bumke-Vogt[2,3], Monika Schreiner[4], Inga Mewis[4], Andrea Borchert[2], Andreas F.H. Pfeiffer[2,3]

[1]Department of Nutrition and Biochemistry, Sciences Faculty-Pontificia Universidad Javeriana Bogota D.C, Colombia; [2]Department of Clinical Nutrition, German Institute of Human Nutrition, Potsdam-Rehbrücke, Nuthetal Germany; [3]Department of Endocrinology, Diabetes and Nutrition, Charité-Universitätsmedizin Berlin, Germany; [4] Department of Quality, Leibniz-Institute of Vegetable and Ornamental Crops Großbeeren/Erfurt e.V., Germany

Keywords: FOXO1, gluconeogenesis, glucose metabolism, isothiocyanates, glucosinolates, MAPKs, BITC, type 2 diabetes.

Background: Type 2 diabetes (T2D) is a health problem found throughout the world. In T2D, an increase in gluconeogenesis and triglyceride synthesis as well as a reduction in fatty acid oxidation accompanied by the presence of reactive oxygen species (ROS) are observed. Altogether, this results in an inappropriate response to insulin. Forkhead box O (FOXO) transcription factors play a crucial role in the regulation of insulin effects on gene expression and metabolism and alterations in FOXO function could contribute to metabolic disorders in diabetes. The consumption of vegetables is related to the prevention of the disease. Nasturtium (*Tropaeolum majus*) possesses high contents of nitrogen sulfur compounds (glucosinolates and isothiocyanates) associated with the prevention of diabetes complications.

Objective: To evaluate the ability of hydrolysed benzyl glucosinolate (BITC) derived from nasturtium to modulate, i) the insulin-signaling pathway, ii) the intracellular localization of FOXO1 and iii) the expression of proteins involved in glucose metabolism, reactive oxygen species detoxification, cell cycle arrest and DNA damage repair.

Methods: The stably transfected human osteosarcoma cells (U-2 OS) with constitutive expression of FOXO1 protein labeled with GFP (green fluorescent protein) were used for FOXO1-GFP visualization by fluorescence microscopy. Life cell images were recorded every minute up to 1 hour for tracing intracellular translocation of FOXO1-GFP after cells treatment with: a) insulin 100 nM; b) BITC 30 to 100 µM and c) insulin + BITC. HepG2 cells were selected to evaluate the effect of BITC on gene and protein expression by the Real-Time quantitative RT-PCR system and Western blotting, respectively.

Results: BITC induced a dose-dependent nuclear translocation of FOXO1-GFP in U-2 OS cells. In HepG2 cells, an inhibition of protein kinase B (AKT/PKB) and FOXO1-phosphorylation was observed. BITC up-regulated the antioxidant and detoxification enzymes Superoxid Dismutase (MnSOD2), Sulfiredoxin 1 (SRXN1), NAD(P)H dehydrogenase (quinone1) (NQO1), and Glutathione peroxidase 2 (GPX2); induced a significant reduction of gluconeogenic enzymes Glucose-6-Phosphatase (G6Pase) and Phosphoenolpyruvate-carboxykinase (PEPCK) and promoted an up-regulation of the cyclin-dependent kinase inhibitor (p21CIP) and Growth Arrest/DNA Damage Repair (GADD45). Except for the nuclear factor (erythroid derived)-like2 (NRF2) and its influence on gene expression of detoxification enzymes, all of the observed effects were independent from FOXO1, AKT and NAD-dependent deacetylase sirtuin-1 (SIRT1) shown by si-RNA knock-down.

Conclusion: Besides an anticarcinogenic potential of isothiocyanates BITC enhances the antioxidative response, promotes longevity and potentially down-regulates the hepatic glucose production, suggesting a role in T2D prevention and treatment.

POSSIBILITY OF EPIGALLOCATECHIN GALLATE AND A-TOCOPHEROL AS FUNCTIONAL FOOD FOR DIABETIC NEPHROPATHY AND THEIR MOLECULAR MECHANISM

Daiki Hayashi[1], Keiko Yagi[2], Shuji Ueda[1], Minoru Yamanoue[1], Hitoshi Ashida[1], Noriaki Emoto[2], Naoaki Saito[3] and Yasuhito Shirai[1]

[1]Department of Agrobioscience, Graduate School of Agricultural Science, and [3]Laboratory of Molecular Pharmacology, Biosignal Research Center, Kobe University, 1-1 Rokkodai, Nada-ku, Kobe 657-8501, Japan; [2]Department of Clinical Pharmacy, Kobe Pharmaceutical University, Japan; Kobe University, Japan

Keywords: Diacylglycerol, protein kinase C, vitamin E, catechin, podocyte

Background: Diabetic nephropathy (DN) is one of the vascular complications of diabetes, causing albuminuria and filtration function failure of the glomerulus. One of the causes for the microvasculature disorder is abnormal protein kinase C (PKC) activation, although any drug and functional food targeting of PKC to prevent and/or improve DN have not been established. Diacylglycerol kinase (DGK) can attenuate PKC activity by converting DG to phosphatidic acid (PA), suggesting that DGK may be a target of functional food to prevent and improve diabetic renal dysfunctions. Indeed, it has been reported that intraperitoneal injection of α-tocopherol (vitamin E; VtE) improved DN by activation of DGK. We also found VtE and epigallocatechin gallate (EGCg) activate DGKα, which is most important DGK subtype involved in the VtE-induced improvement of diabetic nephropathy, through a 67kDa laminin receptor (67LR). However, the molecular mechanism underlying the improvement of nephropathy by intraperitoneal injection of VtE and effects of oral administration of VtE or EGCg on diabetic nephropathy are still unknown.

Objective: The aims of the study are to explore their molecular mechanism underlying the improvement of nephropathy by intraperitoneal injection of VtE and to investigate effects of oral administration of VtE or EGCg on diabetic nephropathy in mice.

Methods: Diabetic mice were produced by intraperitoneal injection of streptozotocin (STZ) using six weeks old male C57BL and DGKα knock out (KO) mice. After confirming the diabetes, the mice were injected VtE () or vehicle every two days. After 6 weeks, the kidney were dissected, and electron microscopy and immunofluorescent staining of DGKα, 67LR, and nephrin were performed. In addition, to investigate effects of oral administration of VtE or EGCg on diabetic nephropathy, the diabetic mice and wild type (WT) were divided into four groups (Control group: non diabetic with normal food, Control+EGCg or VtE group: non diabetic with EGCg or VtE-containing food, STZ group: diabetic mice with normal food, STZ+EGCg or VtE group: diabetic mice with EGCg or VtE food), and we measured urine volume and albumin every week after STZ or vehicle treatment until 6 week. Finally, the mice were sacrificed at end of the experiment and kidney weight was measured.

Results: We found that DGKα and 67LR are colocalized in podocytes in the glomerulus, suggesting their importance of maintenance of podocytes and urinal filter functions. Indeed, VtE treatment protected the disappearance of podocytes during diabetes and improved filter function. Electron microscopic analysis also showed that the VtE treatment rescued diabetic morphological change in the glomerulus. In contrast, the VtE–induced improvement of glomerular morphology and filter function disappeared in the DGKα KO mice. More importantly, oral administration of 0.05 % EGCg and VtE significantly improved the symptoms of diabetic nephropathy.

Conclusion: These results suggest that activation of DGKα by VtE or EGCg protects loss of podocytes during diabetes, contributing maintain the filter function, and that VtE and EGCg may be a good functional food targeting of DGKα to prevent and/or improve diabetic renal dysfunctions.

ASSESSMENT OF CURCUMIN EFFECTS ON ANTIOXIDANTS IN TYPE 2 DIABETIC PATIENTS

Hossein Mirmiranpour [1, 2], **Mehrdad Lari**[2], **Manouchehr Nakhjavani** [2], **Alireza Esteghamati**[2]

[1]Department of Biochemistry, School of Medicine, Alborz University of Medical Sciences, Karaj, Iran, [2]Endocrinology and Metabolism Research Center (EMRC), Vali-Asr Hospital, School of Medicine, Tehran University of Medical Sciences, Tehran, Iran

Keywords: type 2 diabetes mellitus, curcumin, antioxidants, lipid profile

Background: Curcumin, an organic extract of Curcuma, can be useful in the treatment of oxidative stress. It belongs to the family of the rhizomatous herbaceous perennial plant and the coloring agent and food additive properties of this phytochemical plant have been identified. An increase in the antioxidant parameters including FRAP (Ferric Reducing Ability of Plasma), PON 1 (Paraxonase 1), LCAT (Lecithin-cholesterol acyltransferase), LPL (Lipoproteinlipase) connected to lipid profile and GPX (Glutathione peroxidase), SOD (Superoxide dismutase), and Catalase connected to general antioxidant parameters can be implied as inhibitory characters of curcumin on oxidative stress for improving the clinical process of type 2 diabetics. Also, a comparative review between the effect of curcumin on the activity of two recent groups of antioxidant parameters in type 2 diabetes must be considered.

Methods: Serum activities of FRAP, PON 1, LCAT, LPL, GPX, SOD and Catalase belonging to 65, type 2 diabetic patients were analyzed before and after receiving curcumin treatments for 3

months. The activity of the recent parameters was measured using related biochemical methods. Metformin was prescribed to all patients during the mentioned time.

Results: The comparison of antioxidant effects before and after the curcumin therapy showed significantly improved changes after the 3 months study. In such a manner, comparison of the antioxidant effect between the two recent groups of antioxidant parameters after the three month trial significantly demonstrated the most effect of lipid profile depended antioxidant parameters than the other group. Serum activities of FRAP, PON 1, LCAT and LPL of patients after three months were 1363.758 µmol/l (normal range: 612-1634), 67.16743 U/ml (normal range: 5.8-71.13), 36.2768 nmol/ml/hr (normal range: 27.8-38.4) and 26.46237 pmol/ml/hr (normal range: 16.55-29.67) respectively. But the same results for the GPX, SOD and Catalase of patients after the mentioned time were 85.35128 U/ml (normal range: 46.24 - 142.24), 5.274513 U/ml (normal range: 0-10) and 2.564816 U/ml (normal range: 1.3-3.3) respectively (p-value=0.05).

Conclusion: Curcumin can be helpful in the increment of antioxidant activity in type 2 diabetes mellitus. These alterations are remarkable in antioxidant parameters connected to lipid profile.

Part 5
Functional Foods and Neurological Diseases

SOCIOLOGICAL AND ENVIRONMENTAL FACTORS ASSOCIATED WITH MENTAL HEALTH. A FOLLOW UP STUDY OF PATIENTS WITH GERIATRIC DEPRESSION AND COGNITIVE IMPAIRMENT

Carol Dillon, MD, PhD[1,2], Jorge López Camelo, PhD[1], Silvina L. Heisecke, MD[1,2], Fernando E. Taragano, MD, PhD[1,2]

[1]National Scientific and Technical Research Council (CONICET) and [2]SIREN, Department of Neurology, CEMIC University Hospital, Buenos Aires, Argentina

Keywords: Depression, Geriatrics, Prevalence - Incidence - Risk Factors - Causes - Quality of Life - Economic Costs - Follow-up

Background: Sociological factors such as economical burden, caregivers´ burden, gender, and activity, are associated with depression. Depression in older adults is a very common condition that creates a major public health problem. A high percentage of this population is under diagnosed in primary care. The interconnected nature of people and the planet may mean that solutions that benefit both the planet and human health could lie within reach. The concept of planetary health is based on the understanding that human health and human civilization depend on flourishing natural systems and the wise stewardship of those natural systems.

Objectives: The objectives of this work were to: investigate the epidemiology of this disease (causes and risk factors), its implication in cognitive and functional status, quality of life and generated costs. To create a follow up for the patients with geriatric depression associated with cognitive impairment.

Methods: Patients who were consulted for memory problems associated with depression at a memory clinic from a public and a private hospital were recruited during 2005 to 2007. A semi-structured neuropsychiatric interview and an extensive neuropsychological battery with complementary studies were performed.

Results: A hundred and one depressive patients and 25 normal controls were evaluated. There was a significant prevalence and incidence of depression in the geriatric population.

Risk factors: significant differences ($p < 0.05$) compared to normal controls in dyslipidemia, heart disease, cerebrovascular disease, inadequate family support, family history of depression and inactive patients. It was demostrated that inactivity produces a relative risk of 6.5 in developing depression.

Neurological diseases (such as cerebrovascular disease and dementia) become important in the development of depression in this elderly population.

Global cognitive impairment (the majority having subcortical profile) was associated with depression.

Depression caused an alteration in functional status, impaired quality of life and significant health expenditures (such as medical costs).

Results: thirty nine patients (38.6%) were contacted but did not attend the follow-up visits, and sixty one patients were evaluated (61.4%) and followed up. In this last group, only thirty six patients continued with the antidepressant treatment indicated in the baseline visit.

Of the reevaluated patients, 56.6% improved in any area either cognitive or mood. Of the evaluated areas, they were described in mood (anxiety and depression) and into cognitive (memory, attention, executive functions and language) functions. Of these functions, the greatest improvement was observed in depression and anxiety affective spheres. Within the cognitive profile, memory was the most improved cognitive area and secondly attention.

Conclusion: Depression is a prevalent disease in geriatrics. It is important to implement health policies because this disease affects not only the patient but also their environment (family, medical and social system). Health professionals have an essential role in the achievement of planetary health: working across sectors to integrate policies that advance health and environmental sustainability, tackling health inequities, reducing the environmental impacts of health systems, and increasing the resilience of health systems and populations to environmental change.

A 2-YEAR FOLLOW UP STUDY WITH FERMENTED PAPAYA PREPARATION (FPP) MODULATING NOVEL RISK MARKERS OF CARDIOVASCULAR AND NEURODEGENERATIVE DISEASE IN MIDDLE-AGE SUBJECTS WITH IMPENDING METABOLIC SYNDROME.

Francesco Marotta[1], Massimiliano Marcellino[1], Umberto Solimene[2], Biagio Cuffari[3], Aldo Lorenzetti[1], Amelie Mantello[3], Anna Cabeca[4], Oksana Karaushu[1], Joseph Cervi[1], Roberto Catanzaro[3]

[1]ReGenera Research Group for Aging Intervention & Milano Medical, Milano, Italy; [2]WHO-cntr for Traditional Medicine & Biotechnology, University of Milano, Italy; [3]Dept of Internal Medicine, University of Catania, Catania, Italy; [3]Osato Research Institute & Labs, Gifu, Japan; [4]Preventive and Functional Medicine Center, Brunswick, GA, USA;

Keywords: fermented papaya preparation, redox balance, antioxidant, neurodegenerative disease, heavy metals, chelation

Background: In recent years our group has shown that fermented papaya preparation (FPP) (ORI, Oxidative Stress laboratory, Gifu, Japan) on clinical ground could significantly and beneficially affect a number of redox signalling abnormalities in a variety of chronic diseases and as well in age-related markers. In this regard, it has been recently suggested that the aggregation of disease-related proteins in physiological aging can be advocated for by abnormal protein homeostasis. Such abnormalities may thus represent a biomarker of aging affecting life span and being involved in neurodegeneration. As a matter of fact, alpha-synuclein, an aggregation-prone and amyloid-forming protein, has been suggested to play a pivotal role in the pathogenesis of

Parkinson's disease. However, overall, alpha-synuclein and other related markers may have broader implications for healthy aging due to their larger involvement in neuronal plasticity, memory formation overall quality of life patterns. The potential neuroprotective effect of FPP is at the moment the issue of a clinical study on Parkinson's disease patients by the neurology group of Prof. Nordera. This study is showing some preliminary promising results especially in rigidity symptoms and redox biochemistry. Moreover, very recently it has been shown that FPP could dramatically decrease the oxidative stress parameters in Alzheimer's disease (AD) patients. (Barbagallo M et al 2015).

Objective: To review the latest achievements of FPP integrative treatment of neurodegenerative disease while, at the same time, presenting the final data of a 2-year trial using FPP in patients with impending metabolic disease bearing a higher risk to develop a neurodegenerative disease too.

Methods: Exclusion criteria were; secondary hypertension, cardiomyopathy, severe abnormalities of liver and kidney function, cerebrovascular diseases, grossly elevated total cholesterol (>280mg/dl or LDL >180mg/dl), malignancies and history of coronary bypass surgery or on insulin treatment were excluded from this study. Exclusion criteria were also the consumption of antioxidant or other supplements. Ninety-four subjects ranging from 45 to 66 years old, with impending metabolic syndrome (mild features of hypertension, insulin resistance, dyslipidemia) were included. All were screened for ApoE level to rule out risk gene pattern. This was a RCT, double-blind, with FPP 4.5g given twice a day vs common antioxidant cocktail (trans-resveratrol 10mg, selenium 60mcg, vit E 10mg, vit C 50mg) for 9 months. Then, after two weeks wash-out period, a treatment was restarted by adding heavy a chabasite-phillipsite-based silicates which occur in nature, CellularDetox-chelator, 3gr at bedtime for further 12 weeks and biochemical tests were re-done. At the end of this period, the original FPP and antioxidant cocktail schedule was resumed and maintained for further 12 months. All procedures were approved by an independent Ethical Committee for nonpharmacological research. Each subject recruited for the study was fully informed and treated in compliance with the guidelines of the Declaration of Helsinki. Parameters included: cyclophilin-A, oxidative stress, plasminogen activator inhibitor-1, anti-oxidised LDL and faecal excretion of heavy metals, recently pointed out as co-factors of neurodegenerative diseases. Other common biomarkers have been tested as well.

Results: The data of our study confirmed that FPP seems to decrease not only oxidative stress parameters ($p < 0.05$ vs antioxidant cocktail mixture) but, unlike the control antioxidant, it did uniquely decrease also oxidised-LDL ($p < 0.01$ vs baseline and vs antioxidant cocktail mixture), although unaffecting the lipid profile per sè. Moreover, only FPP decreased cyclophilin-A plasma level and plasminogen activator-inhibitor ($p < 0.05$ vs antioxidant cocktail mixture). Insulin resistance was only slight but not significantly improved. Heavy metal gut clearance was not affected by any of the nutraceuticals. However, this CellularDetox-chelator, by itself remarkably increased fecal gut discharge of heavy metals but only in those patients with abnormal baseline values ($p < 0.001$ vs baseline). The addition of chelator to the control nutraceuticals didn't prove to yield better results while the addition to FPP showed a trend increase of the discharge of aluminum and cadmium ($p < .0.05$ vs oral chelator alone).

Conclusion: The damage caused by oxidative stress is one of the earliest pathophysiological events in the development of endothelial dysfunction and in neurodegenerative diseases and the brain is characterized by a low content of antioxidant systems. Identification and application of such biomarkers in nutritional and life-style interventional plans may help influence or, ideally, prevent concomitant illnesses. Our preliminary data suggest that FPP might play a significant role within a comprehensive preventive medicine strategy plan for impending metabolic diseases and potentially associated neurodegenerative disease. Effective heavy metal chelators remains a further additive avenue to possibly pursue in consideration of the reports linking neurodegenerative disease and long term subtle heavy metal accumulation at brain level. It is likely that a longer term pollutant chelation together with effective redox-modulators such as FPP may prove to be a promising strategy to apply in larger cohort of subjects. This holds of interest when considering that an uncontrolled supplementation of high dosages of random vitamins has to be discouraged (Sax JK.Am J Law Med. 2015) but also taking into account the failure of high dosages of fruit and vegetable in significantly bring about a beneficial modification of redox system (TE Crane, J Nutr 2011) or upregulating key DNA-protecting genes (Møller P, Cancer Epidemiol Biomarkers Prev. 2003).

BODY MASS, METABOLIC AND CARDIOVASCULAR IMPACT OF AQUATIC EXERCISE AND NUTRITIONAL GUIDANCE FOR INDIVIDUALS WITH CHRONIC INCOMPLETE SPINAL CORD INJURY (CMISCI)

William H. Scott, Joanne E Smith, Kylie James, Peter H. Gorman, Paula Richley Geigle

University of Maryland Rehabilitation and Orthopaedic Institute, Baltimore, Maryland, USA

Keywords: spinal cord injury, nutrition, weight gain, obesity, insulin resistance, metabolic changes, glucose, insulin and A1C

Background: After sustaining spinal cord injury (SCI) there are numerous factors contributing to weight gain (as a result over 65% of people with SCI are overweight). Factors include; changes in body composition with a loss of lean muscle mass due to loss of nerve innervation, and increased fat mass; people with SCI experience interrupted neural connectivity to musculoskeletal system which lowers metabolic rates from pre-injury rates; some medications, such as narcotics, also potentially decrease resting metabolic rates; reduced physical activity results in decreased energy output and calories burned reduction of 12 to 54% total daily energy expenditure; many people with SCI continue to eat the same portion sizes/calories as pre-injury despite drop in RMR; hormonal changes occur with decreased growth hormone and testosterone associated with lean tissue mass loss and an increase in fat gaining hormones, insulin and cortisol; glucose intolerance and poor carbohydrate metabolism. A decrease in lean muscle mass and increase in adipose tissue after SCI can impair glucose uptake. In particular problems occur with carbohydrate metabolism, therefore carbohydrates -grains and starchy vegetables - need to be limited.

Objectives: Assess dosed group aquatic exercise at 70-75% of heart rate reserve (HRR) and nutritional guidance upon body mass, glucose, insulin, A1C, peak VO_2, and resting metabolic rate (RMR) for three individuals with CMISCI and fasting glucose greater than 100 mg/dL.

Participants/methods: Four men: 63 yo, AIS D, body mass index (BMI) 31.9; 34 yo who is non ambulatory, AIS C, BMI of 31.6; 58 yo, AIS D, BMI 27.4 and 45 yo who is non ambulatory, AIS C, BMI of 30.9. We prescribed dosed aquatic exercise program 3 times per week for 10 weeks, and a weekly phone nutritional consult by phone. Nutritional guidance included reducing refined carbohydrates and processed food, limiting high glycemic fruits, and increasing vegetable, fluid and lean protein intake. Outcome measures (pre/post) included: three-day electronic food logs, weekly hard copy food logs, glucose, insulin and A1C (via standard fasting venipuncture), peak VO_2 and RMR.

Results: Participant one decreased glucose, 20% (132 to 106 mg/dL); A1C, 11% (6.3-5.6); weight, 10%, (11.9 kg); RMR, 13%; and peak VO_2, 12%; participant two increased glucose, 9%; A1C, no change; decreased weight, 3% (3.3 kg); decreased peak VO2, 18.5 RMR, 4.5%; participant three decreased: glucose, 14%, (126 to 108 mg/dL); A1C, 5% (7.5 to 7.1); weight, 6% (88.9 to 83.8 kg); and increased peak VO_2, 8% (21.9 to 23.7) and RMR, 12.5%; participate four decreased: A1C, 5.5% (5.5 to 5.2); weight, 0.7% (106.4 to 105.7 kg); and increased glucose, 9.3%, (86 to 94 mg/dL); peak VO_2, 34.1% (11.9 to 16) and RMR, 24.6%.

Goal: (-) intake; (+) intake	201 pre	201 post	Δ	202 pre	202 post	Δ	203 pre	203 post	Δ	204 pre	204 post	Δ
Calories (-)	1980	1101		1810	932		1009	1159	+150	2221	1332	
Calories from fat (-)	702	381		716	327		531	361		701	421	
Carbohydrates (-)	224	104		189	84		68	132	+64	306	184	
Fiber (+)	20	12	-8	7	16		17	11	-6	17	10	-7
Total Sugars (-)	96	62		70	11		21	91	+70	113	67	
Fat (-)	78	42		79	36		59	40		78	46	
Saturated fat (-)	26	15		16	8		15	9		21	12	
Water (+)	1113	1243		2306	2431		471	1292		1134	680	-454
Protein (+)	103	80	-23	83	65	-18	54	79		74	44	-30

Conclusion: Moderate exercise with weekly nutritional guidance decreased body mass, glucose, and A1C in two out of three CMISCI individuals. Further examination of the impact a low cost intervention of combined aquatic exercise with nutritional guidance exerts upon body mass, metabolic status, and cardiovascular fitness for individuals with CMISCI is indicated.

VITAMIN B12 SUPPLEMENTATION AND COGNITIVE SCORES IN GERIATRIC PATIENTS HAVING MILD COGNITIVE IMPAIRMENT

Komal Chauhan[1] and Aditika Agarwal[1]

[1]Department of Foods and Nutrition, The Maharaja Sayajirao University of Baroda, Vadodara- 390002 Gujarat, India

Keywords: Mild Cognitive Impairment, vitamin B12, geriatrics, cognition

Background: Neurodegenerative diseases are increasingly affecting the elderly with severe impact on their brain health. There is a wide gap in the supplementation based studies for increasing the cognition levels of the geriatric population especially in the developing countries like India, which are at extreme risk for having neurological disorders. The vitamin B12 herein has lately caught much attention for improving the cognitive status. The literature has linked the possibility of alleviating neurological disorders in the elderly with the effective vitamin B12 management. The abundant animal and human models have proved that supplementation of vitamin B12 is beneficial for restoration of the cognitive functions.

Objective: To supplement the vitamin B12 deficient Mild Cognitively Impaired (MCI) geriatric patients with the vitamin B12 injectable doses and impact evaluation.

Methods: The screening of the MCI patients was done through the Mini-Mental State Examination and Yamaguchi Fox Pigeon Imitation test. Baseline information was elicited from the patients residing in urban Vadodara (a district in the state of Gujarat), India. This included socio-demographic, medical and drug history, anthropometric, physical activity pattern and biochemical parameters comprising of serum vitamin B12 and glycated haemoglobin profile. The sub-sample of 60 patients with MCI demonstrating severe vitamin B12 deficiency were conveniently enrolled for of Vitamin B_{12} 1000 µg injectable doses in dosage of 1,000 µg every day for one week, followed by 1,000 µg every week for 4 weeks & then 1,000 µg for remaining 4 months. Post six months intervention the entire parameters were elicited.

Results: The vitamin B12 supplementation resulted in a significant (p<0.001) improvement in the MMSE scores of the patients with a rise of 9.63% in the total patients. The gender-wise division also highlighted a significant increase (p<0.001) in the scores by 6.79% and 12.46% in males and females whereas 10.20% and 8.24% for young-old (60-69 yrs) and old-old (70-85 yrs) categories respectively. As a result, 27 patients progressed towards the normal category from the MCI state being assessed by MMSE scores. In the same manner, YGFPIT too demonstrated a 38% normal increase with 35% males, 42% females, 41% young–old and 31% old-old moving to normal status. Thus, a number of 28 patients progressed to normal condition as per YGFPIT.

Conclusion: Hence, vitamin B12 supplementation was significantly effective in placing the serum vitamin B12 of MCI patients from deficiency state to sufficient levels and in turn increased their performance in MMSE and YFPIT scores.

NEUROPROTECTIVE EFFECTS OF PHYTOESTROGENS DERIVED FROM *FLEMINGIA STROBILIFERA* VIA ENHANCING NEUROGLOBIN EXPRESSION

Si-Yeon Jeong [1], Minsun Chang [2], Sangho Choi [3], Sei-Ryang Oh [4], Zhanyang Yu [5], Xiaoying Wang [5], and Yun Seon Song [1]

[1]College of Pharmacy, Sookmyung Women's University, Seoul 140-742, Republic of Korea; [2]Department of Biosystems, Sookmyung Women's University, Seoul 140-742, Republic of Korea; [3]International Biological Material Research Center, KRIBB, Daejeon 305-806, Republic of Korea; [4]Natural Medicine Research Center, KRIBB, ChungBuk, 363-883, Republic of Korea; [5]Neuroprotection Research Laboratory, Departments of Neurology and Radiology, Massachusetts General Hospital, 149 13th Street, Charlestown, MA 02129, USA.

Keywords: *Flemingia strobilifera*, Phytoestrogen, Estrogen receptor, MCF-7 cell, Uterus, Neuroglobin, Neuroprotection

Background: Phytoestrogen has received attention due to its high neuroprotective efficacy and safety for aged women. To elucidate the effect of phytoestrogen in aged female, we first identified an estrogenic property of *Flemingia strobilifera* (FS) and found several phytoestrogens in *Flemingia strobilifera* extract (FSE). Recently, it has also been reported that phytoestrogen shows neuroprotective properties through upregulation of neuroglobin (Ngb), a tissue globin in the brain.

Objective: This study aims to discover neuroprotective effect of phytoestrogens derived from FSE, which is mediated by Ngb upregulation *in vitro* as well as *in vivo*.

Methods: We determined the estrogenic activity of FSE using estrogen receptor (ER) binding, estrogen response element (ERE)

promoter transcriptional activity, which was confirmed by gene expression as well as cell proliferation. Estrogenic property was also tested in immature female rats. To identify active estrogenic compounds (phytoestrogens) from FSE, we used NMR, HPLC and MS. Furthermore we examined the neuroprotective effect mediated by Ngb upregulation of FSE and phytoestrogens. This was achieved using Ngb promoter activity assay, qPCR, and LDH assay. Behavior tests consisting of open field, elevated plus maze, tail suspension, and forced swimming tests were conducted on both young and aged mice.

Results: Estrogenic activity of FSE was discovered, and five phytoestrogens (compound 1-5) were identified. FSE, compound 1, 2, 4 and 5 showed binding affinities for recombinant human estrogen receptor alpha (hERα) with IC_{50} of 10^{-7} M to 10^{-5} M. FSE, compound 1 and 5 also activated ERE transcription in MCF-7 cell with EC_{50} of 10^{-6} M ($p < 0.05$, $p < 0.05$, respectively). In addition, FSE and compounds 1-5 induced MCF-7 cell proliferation at 10^{-5} M and of trefoil factor 1 (pS2) mRNA expression ($p < 0.001$). In immature female rats, a significant uterine weight increase was noted in FSE treated rats without body weight gain ($p < 0.001$). Interestingly protein expression of ERα in uteri decreased ($p < 0.01$) while the protein expressions of PR-A and PR-B increased significantly in FSE treated rats ($p < 0.001$). The pS2 gene expressions in FSE treated rat uteri were slightly up-regulated. Furthermore, neuroprotective effects of FSE and compound 1-3 were determined by observing increased levels of Ngb promoter activity in SKNSH and N2a cells ($p < 0.001$, $p < 0.05$, respectively). Up-regulation of Ngb was then confirmed in mRNA level. In FSE concentration of $5x10^{-7}$ g/ml to 10^{-5} g/ml, cell cytotoxicity induced by hydrogen peroxide was reduced ($p < 0.05$). In aged female mouse brain, FSE increased Ngb protein levels. Lastly, FSE decreased times in corner in the open field test and the number of closed arm entries in the elevated plus maze tests. On the other hand FSE increased the mobility time in the tail suspension and the latency time in the passive avoidance tests. It indicated that FSE ameliorated anxiety, depression and cognitive impairment in aged female mice.

Conclusion: In this present study, we identified the estrogenic activity of FSE and five phytoestrogens (compound 1-5). Furthermore we elucidated the neuroprotective effect of FSE and its compounds mediated by Ngb upregulation. Our result suggests that phytoestrogens derived from FSE are promising candidates for Ngb-targeted neuroprotective therapy in aged women.

CHARNOLY BODY AS A NOVEL BIOMARKER OF NUTRITIONAL STRESS IN ALZHEIMER'S DISEASE

Sushil Sharma, Joseph Choga, Vineet Gupta, Pearl Doghor, Ankur Chauhan, Fredy Kalala, Alison Foor, Christopher Wright, James Renteria, Krystel Elliott-Theberge, Shubhra Mathur

Saint James School of Medicine, Cane Hall, St Vincent, St Vincent & Grenadines

Keywords: Charnoly Body, Nutrition, Metallothioneins, Cortisol, IGF-1, BDNF, Alzheimer's disease

Background: Charnoly body (CB) was discovered initially in the developing undernourished rat cerebellar Purkinje neurons and in the *Domoic Acid- as Kainic Acid, Acromelic Acid, PCBs, Lead, Arsenic, and Mercury* exposed mice hippocampal and hypothalamic neurons. The incidence of CB is increased with the severity of nutritional and environmental neurotoxic insult. We reported CB as a universal biomarker of cell injury in nanomedicine and chronic drug addiction. Subsequently, CB was detected in various cellular and animal models of fetal alcohol syndrome, Parkinson's disease, Alzheimer's disease, vascular dementia, chronic drug addiction, and during intrauterine exposure to environmental neurotoxins.

Objective: We have now proposed that stress (nutritional/environmental)-induced cortisol release augments, whereas metallothioneins (MTs), IGF-1, and BDNF inhibit hippocampal CB formation to prevent progressive neurodegeneration, and hence early morbidity and mortality in AD.

Methods: Early events in CB formation including: $\Delta\Psi$ collapse, down-regulation of mitochondrial ubiquinone-NADH-oxidoreductase (Complex-1), which serves as a rate-limiting enzyme complex for the mitochondrial electron transport chain for ATP synthesis, and 8-OH-2dG can be detected in the blood, saliva, semen, and urine samples as CB rudiments to evaluate epigenetic modulation of DNA methylation and histone acetylation following neuronal injury. During chronic phase, CB can be detected at the ultrastructure level in the neurons, platelets, lymphocytes, cells of the buccal mucosa, skin cells, oocyte, spermatocyte, and in any highly vulnerable cell. The incidence of CB formation was increased and neuritogenesis was attenuated as a function of nutritional stress and in the mitochondrial genome knock out (RhO$_{mgko}$) human dopaminergic (SK-N-SH, SHS-Y-5Y) neurons due to down-regulation of the rate limiting enzyme, complex-1. Transfection of aging RhO$_{mgko}$ neurons with the gene encoding complex-1, inhibited CB formation and augmented neuritogenesis in this cellular model of aging, as we discovered in gene-manipulated α-Synuclein-metallothioneins triple knock out and weaver mutant (wv/wv) mice as animal models of neurodegeneration, AD, PD, and multiple drug abuse respectively. The brain regional CB formation was attenuated in MTs-over-expressing weaver mutant (wv/wv-MTs) mice as an animal model of nutritional and drug rehabilitation.

Results: At the ultrastructural level, CB appears as a pleomorphic, electron-dense multi-lamellar, quasi-crystalline, stack of degenerated mitochondrial membranes, causing progressive neurodegeneration in highly vulnerable neurons of the aging brain and may be induced by *viral* infection during intrauterine life from infected parents.

CB is a pre-apoptotic biomarker of compromised mitochondrial bioenergetics and is formed in response to nutritional stress, intrauterine infection, environmental toxins, and/or drugs of abuse due to free radical overproduction and mitochondrial genome down-regulation.

Accumulation of CB at the junction of axon hillock impairs axoplasmic transport of various enzymes, neurotransmitters, hormones, neurotropic factors (NGF, BDNF), and mitochondria at the synaptic terminals to cause cognitive impairment, early morbidity, and mortality. Nonspecific induction of CB induces alopecia, myelosuppression, and GIT symptoms in multi-drug-resistant malignancies.

Antioxidants and neurotropic growth factors such as MTs inhibited CB formation as free radical scavengers by activating zinc-mediated transcriptional regulation of genes involved in growth, proliferation, differentiation, and development. Hence novel drugs may be developed to prevent CB formation or enhance charnolophagy as a basic molecular mechanism of intracellular detoxification during acute phase, and CB antagonists to avert cognitive impairments in AD by employing CB as an early, sensitive and specific biomarker.

Conclusion: Based on two types of monoamine oxidases on the outer mitochondrial membranes, we have proposed two types of CBs (i.e MOA-specific CB, and MOA-B-specific CB), which can be targeted *in vivo* by ^{11}C or ^{18}F-labeled monoamine oxidase-A or B inhibitors to detect CB formation in the aging AD brain, in addition of ^{18}FdG-PET neuroimaging to assess the mitochondrial bioenergetics in AD.

A DIETARY PORTFOLIO MODULATES SIRT1 EXPRESSION IN ASTROCYTES AND REDUCES BRAIN INFLAMMATION WHILE IMPROVING WORKING MEMORY IN A TRANSGENIC MICE MODEL OF ALZHEIMER DISEASE.

Syeda Tauqeerunnisa Begum[1], Ana Laura Pinedo Vargas [2], Sofia Diaz-Cintra[2], Nimbe Torres Y Torres[3], Claudia Perez-Cruz[1]

[1]Department of Pharmacology, Centro de Investigación y de Estudios Avanzados, del Instituto Politécnico Nacional, Mexico City; [2]UNAM-Institute of Neurobiology Juriquilla, Mexico; [3]Instituto Nacional de Ciencias Médicas y de la Nutricion, Mexico City

Keywords: Alzheimer's disease, neuroinflammation, synapsis, SIRT1, bioactive food

Background: Alzheimer's disease (AD) is the most common form of dementia that involves neurodegenerative processes affecting synaptic function and memory formation. Recent investigations have described brain metabolic alteration in early stages of AD, such as a hypo metabolism of glucose, brain insulin resistance and reduced mitochondrial bioenergetics. Astrocytes function as key components on brain metabolism and can protect against oxidative stress; however, in AD there is an over activation of astrocytes that leads to inflammatory reactions and neuronal damage. Sirtuin 1 (SIRT1) has emerged as a key metabolic sensor in various cellular processes. SIRT1 mediates mitochondrial biogenesis, while suppresses the expression of pro-inflammatory cytokines by astrocytes. Functional foods contain bioactive components that can modulate expression and function of proteins and enzymes related to energy metabolism. A dietary portfolio (PD) containing dried nopal, chía seed, and soy was able to restore metabolic disturbances in obese subjects (Guevara-cruz et al., 2012), while nopal reduced neuroinflammation, APP levels, oxidative stress, and increased synaptic contacts in obese rats (Leonhardt et al., 2014). Moreover, food may have epigenetic effects and may accelerate or delay the progression of disease (Martin et al., 2013, Martin et al., 2014). Therefore, we aim to evaluate in 3xTgAD mice (AD transgenic animal model) whether ingestion of a PD over two generations may increase SIRT1 expression in astrocytes and principal neurons. We hypothesize that 3xTgAD mice fed with a PD will present higher levels of SIRT1 in astrocytes, reduced neuroinflammation, and improved cognitive abilities compared to transgenic mice fed with control chow diet.

Objective: 1. To evaluate the expression of SIRT1 in astrocytes on first and second generation of female 3xTgAD mice fed with a PD and compared with 3xTgAD and non-transgenic (non-Tg) mice fed with control diet. 2. To evaluate the amount of GFAP positive neurons and the cognitive performance of 3xTgAD mother and female offspring fed with a PD and compare to controls.

Method: 3xTgAD and age matched wild type female mice will be fed with either control diet (AIN-93) or PD over two subsequent generations. Cognitive performance will be asses at 9 months-old by the T-maze and water maze before sacrifice. Whole cell and synaptic extracts will be used to asses SIRT1, Pgc-1, PAAR γ, Bdnf, Irisin, Arc and Psd-95 by Western Blot. Double immunofluorescence was used to confirm the presence of SIRT on GFAP positive cells (astrocytes) and dendritic processes were analyzed under laser confocal microscopy (Leica SP-8).

Results: Nine-months old 3XTgAD female mice fed with PD had an improved spatial and working memory compared to AIN-93 fed 3xTgAD mice. This was accompanied by decrease inflammation in hippocampus and altered regional distribution of SIRT1 in astrocytic processes. In addition, synaptic proteins were enhanced in mice 3xTgAD mice fed with PD.

Conclusion: Nutritional strategies have been proposed as therapeutic alternatives for degenerative diseases, and may modulate the course of Alzheimer´s disease. The portfolio dietary used in the present study, improved some markers of energy metabolism, while rescue memory performance and alleviates neuroinflammation in AD transgenic mice.

Part 6
Functional Foods and Cardiovascular Diseases (CVD)

THE EFFECTS OF FUNCTIONAL FOOD ON REHABILITATION OF CORONARY HEARTS DISEASE PATIENTS

Alexander Plakida [1], Elena Usenko [2], Tamara Zhuravl'ova [2]

[1]Odessa National Medical University, Odessa, Ukraine, [2]PI Ukrainian Scientific Research Institute of Medical Rehabilitation and Resort Therapy of the Ministry of Health of Ukraine, Odessa, Ukraine

Keywords: functional food, coronary heart disease, obesity, lipid metabolism, sanatorium treatment.

Background: Patients with coronary heart disease (CHD) are at high cardiovascular risk (CWR), due to a complex set of inter-related hemodynamic, metabolic and neurohormonal disorders. Particular importance is the correction of body weight as one of the most modifiable risk factors. The connecting link between the risk of coronary heart disease and obesity is dyslipidemia. The use of pharmaceutical products helps to improve the results of treatment of CHD, however, drug therapy has a number of disadvantages, the main of which are allergic reactions, development of addiction, side effects. Rehabilitation treatment of patients with CVD in the sanatorium stage provides for the mandatory inclusion of non-drug interventions, such as physical therapy and dietetics. One of the promising directions of currently research of correction of weight is the use of functional foods. We have received positive results in preliminary studies in athletes by use of functional foods containing L-carnitine. On this basis, we have developed a functional product for patients with CVD taking into account the peculiarities of metabolism.

Objective: To investigate the efficacy of functional foods in patients with CVD at the stage of sanatorium treatment for weight loss and normalization of lipid metabolism

Methods: 30 patients with CHD FC I-II, 14 men, 16 women, mean age - (52,2 ± 2,4), were divided into 2 groups: a control received the standard range of spa treatments, while the main additionally received 2 types of functional food. The first, "LFK-1" included L-carnitine, taurine, inositol, choline, coenzyme Q_{10}, was held for 15-20 minutes before the start of gymnastic exercises. Second, "LFK-3", for correction of psycho-emotional status included vitamins A, B2, E, B5, B6, B12, PP, D, C, extracts of motherwort, hawthorn, valerian, succinic acid, chromium was carried out for 15-20 minutes before a night's sleep. The duration of treatment was 21 days. Investigations, before and after the courses, included: anamnesis, dynamic clinical observation of objective and subjective condition, laboratory diagnostics (general clinical research, lipidogram, coagulogram, liver function tests, transaminase), instrumental methods of investigation (measurement of blood pressure (BP), electrocardiogram (ECG) in 12 standard leads, Holter ECG monitoring, assessment of quality of life (WHO questionnaire WHOQOL-100). The body mass composition was investigated by using body composition monitor "Omron" BF-511.

Results: After a course of spa treatment, in the main group showed a significant reduction ($p < 0.001$) in body weight, which led to a similar decrease in body mass index. It should be noted a significant decrease in the absolute content of fat components of body composition. At the same time, there was a decrease in total level of cholesterol from (7,2±0,38) to (5,8±0,31) mM/l ($p < 0.001$) and triglycerides from (3,4±0,28) to (2,2±0,26) mM/l ($p < 0.001$). In both groups there was a significant positive dynamics of the degree of reduction of PC in patients with coronary heart disease after a course of SCR. In the study group, the degree of reduction of PC was decreased by 1.8 times ($p < 0.05$), while in the control group treated with the standard, set of the degree of reduction of PC decreased by 1.3 times ($p < 0.05$). The improvement of the clinical course of the underlying disease, the degree of reduction of cardiovascular risk in the form of lower body mass index, the improvement of clinical and laboratory parameters and increase of physical capacity of patients with coronary artery disease accompanied by positive dynamics of the main indicators of quality of life.

Conclusion: Our study demonstrated that the use of functional foods in patients with CVD significantly reduced body weight and fat components, normalize lipid metabolism and improves exercise tolerance.

HISTOPATHOLOGICAL ASSESSMENT OF THE CARDIOPROTECTIVE INFLUENCE OF *CAULERPA LENTILLIFERA* CRUDE LIPID EXTRACT AGAINST THE DEVELOPMENT OF ISOPROTERENOL-INDUCED MYOCARDIAL INJURY IN A MURINE MODEL

R. J. B. Simbulan[1], P. E. E. Calderon[1,2], R. A. Layug[1], A. B. P. Al-os[1], J. R. J. Go[1], M. E. C. Goco[1], K. T. M. Javar[1], D. F. Labiano[1], D. K. S. Parde[1], A. G. A. Perez[1], I. J. Y. Rodriguez[1], A. F. Santos III[1], N. L. Sergio[1], J. E. M. Sincioco[1], and M. A. P. Tiangco[1]

[1]College of Medicine, San Beda College, 638 Mendiola Street, San Miguel, Manila, Philippines; [2]Biology Department, College of Science, De La Salle University, 2401 Taft Avenue, Manila, Philippines

Keywords: myocardial infarction, isoproterenol, *Caulerpa lentillifera*, crude lipid extract, cardioprotective effect

Background: Cardiovascular disease (CVD) is the leading cause of mortality in the Philippines and in the world. Each year, more people die of CVDs than any other cause. In the Philippines, coronary heart disease (CHD)-related deaths reached around 14% of the total deaths nationwide. *Caulerpa lentillifera* (Bryopsidales: Caulerpaceae), an edible seaweed locally cultivated in southeast Asia, is known for its many health benefits and may perhaps be a potential food source for cardioprotection. In an effort to investigate the benefits of functional foods and natural products in possibly reducing CVD-related morbidity and mortality, this study was conducted as a pilot investigation on the cardioprotective influence of the crude lipid extract of *C. lentillifera* against the development of myocardial infarction (MI) in an animal model.

Objectives: To evaluate the effects of oral supplementation with *C. lentillifera* crude lipid extract (CLE) on cardiac histology of adult Sprague-Dawley rats with isoproterenol (ISO)-induced MI. Specifically, the following were determined: (1) the phytochemical constituents of CLE and (2) the effects of CLE on histopathologic changes in the myocardial fibers, edema, and inflammatory cell infiltration in experimental myocardial infarction.

Methods: Crude lipid extract of *C. lentillifera* was obtained using a modified Folch method and was analyzed using gas chromatography-mass spectrometry (GC-MS). Thirty (30) eight-week old, male Sprague-Dawley rats were randomized to four treatment groups: (1) sham group (plain normal saline solution [PNSS] only), (2) ISO control group, (3) CLE control group (CLE+PNSS), and (4) experimental group (CLE+ISO). Oral pre-treatment with CLE was done for 17 days via gastric gavage. ISO control and CLE+ISO groups were given single doses of ISO (85 mg/kg/dose) subcutaneously on the 18th and 19th days (24 hours apart) to induce MI. Immediately following the second dose of ISO, the hearts were excised under the supervision of a licensed veterinarian who was blinded to the study. Histopathological examination of the left ventricular wall was done under light microscopy. The extent of myocardial damage, edema and inflammation was evaluated using a standard numerical scheme. Data analysis employed Kruskal-Wallis tests to compare the extent of tissue injury among the groups, followed by Mann-Whitney U tests with Bonferroni correction.

Results: Phytochemical screening of CLE showed the presence of linoleic acid [18:2 (*n*-6)], palmitic acid [16:0], stearic acid [18:0], oleic acid [18:1 (*n*-9)], and β-sitosterol (β-sitosterin). There was no mortality in any of the subjects during and post-induction of MI. Results showed normal cardiac tissue (median grade 0) in the sham and CLE groups, while there was extensive myocardial injury (median grade 3) in the ISO group, described as necrosis with diffuse inflammation. This confirmed the histopathologic diagnosis of MI in the ISO group. The CLE-treated group showed less severe MI (median grade 2), described as extensive myofibrillar degeneration with or without diffuse inflammation. When compared to the ISO control, the CLE+ISO group showed marked reduction in the incidence of myocardial injury ($p<0.05$).

Table 1. **Histopathological Assessment of Cardiac Tissue Injury (MI)**

Treatment Group	Median Histologic Grade	Incidence of MI (%)			
		Grade 0	Grade 1	Grade 2	Grade 3
Sham (n=8)	0	100	0	0	0
ISO control (n=7)	3	0	0	28.6	71.4
CLE control (n=8)	0	72.5	15	12.5	0
ISO+CLE (n=7)	2	0	28.6	71.4	0

Conclusion: Phytochemical analysis of CLE demonstrated the presence of linoleic acid [18:2 (n-6)], palmitic acid [16:0], stearic acid [18:0], oleic acid [18:1 (n-9)], and β-sitosterol (β-sitosterin), components believed to possess potential cardioprotective properties. There was significant attenuation of the development of MI in the CLE-treated groups. These findings suggest that CLE may have potential cardioprotective influence against the development of myocardial injury in this animal model of MI.

EFFECT OF RESVERATROL ON ENDOTHELIAL CELLS INCUBATED WITH PLASMA FROM PREECLAMPSIA WOMEN (*IN VITRO* MODEL)

Valeria Cristina Sandrim[1], Mayara Dias-Caldeira[1], Jose Sergio Possonato-Vieira[1], Ricardo Cavalli[2]

[1]Departmento de Farmacologia, Instituto de Biociências, Universidade Estadual Paulista (UNESP), Botucatu, São Paulo, Brazil; [2]Departmento de Ginecologia e Obstetricia, Faculdade de Medicina de Ribeirao Preto, Universidade de Sao Paulo (FMRP-USP), Ribeirao Preto, Brazil

Keywords: resveratrol, nitric oxide, preeclampsia, endothelial cells

Background: Preeclampsia (PE) is the main cause of mother and fetus mortality worldwide. It is characterized by hypertension in pregnancy accompanied of proteinuria, and woman who develops PE has increase risk to develop cardiovascular diseases posteriorly. It is well evidenced that nitric oxide (NO) bioavailability is reduced in preeclampsia compared to healthy pregnant. Resveratrol is a polyphenolic compound presented in high quantity in red wine that stimulates endothelial nitric oxide synthesis (eNOS, enzyme that synthesizes NO in endothelial cells). Based on two-stage model of preeclampsia (placental ischemia and endothelial dysfunction), we are exploring an *in vitro* model of preeclampsia, which consist of the incubation of plasma from pregnant (with preeclampsia and respective control) with endothelial cell cultures.

Objective: To verify if resveratrol induces more production of NO and improve cell viability in endothelial cells incubated with plasma from preeclampsia and healthy pregnant.

Methods: We collected blood from matched (age, BMI, race and non-smoker) healthy pregnant (HP, n=5) and preeclampsia (PE, n=5). Blood was centrifuged and plasma was incubated (10% v/v) for 24 hours in endothelial cells (HUVECs, ATCC's cell line: CRL 2873) with (+R) or not (-R) 30 μM trans-resveratrol. Cellular viability was measured using MTT assay and nitric oxide was measured by quantification of nitrite (NO metabolite) by following technique: 50 μL of cell supernatant were placed in 96 well plate added with 50 μL of sulfanilamide (1% in acidic solution) and incubated for 10 minutes. Then, 50 μL of N-(1-Naphthyl) ethylene diamine dihydrochloride (NED) solution 5% were added and plate was incubated for another 10 minutes. Plate was read in spectrophotometer (Biotek, Synergy4) in 540nm. We used ANOVA and the Bonferroni post-test to verify differences among groups. P value < 0.05 was considered statistically different.

Results: Regarding MTT, in both group (HP and PE), resveratrol reduced cell proliferation when compared with cultures without resveratrol (reduction of 60% in HP and 20% in PE); moreover, no differences were found comparing HP vs PE neither in –R cultures nor +R (all P>0.05). Interestingly regarding nitrite levels, we found that cultures incubated with plasma from PE presented reduced levels of nitrite compared to cultures incubated with plasma from HP (5.6 ± 2.0 μM vs 1.0 ± 0.13 μM, P<0.05). When resveratrol was added (+R cultures), no differences were found comparing cultures incubated with HP plasma with (+R) or without (–R) resveratrol (6.2 ± 2.7 μM vs 5.6 ± 2.0 μM, P>0.05). However, in cultures incubated with plasma from PE, we found significant differences (increase of 60%) comparing nitrite produced in +R cultures compared to –R cultures (1.6 ± 0.45 μM vs 1.0 ± 0.13 μM, respectively, P<0.05).

Conclusion: Our study demonstrates that resveratrol improved NO production in an in vitro model of preeclampsia. Moreover, cultures incubated with plasma from PE pregnant show reduced NO production compared to HP, which consolidates literature evidences. Therefore, our results suggest that a diet rich in resveratrol, such as red grape juice, could be indicated to preeclampsia women. This study was funded by the Conselho Nacional de Desenvolvimento Cientifico e Tecnologico (CNPq-Brazil) and by the Fundação de Amparo a Pesquisa do Estado de São Paulo (FAPESP-Brazil).

Part 7
Functional Foods and Cancer

GREEN TEA POLYPHENOL INDUCES CHANGES IN CANCER-RELATED FACTORS IN AN ANIMAL MODEL OF BLADDER CANCER

Akihiro Asai[1], Yasuyoshi Miyata[1], Tomohiro Matsuo[1], Kojiro Ohba[1], Yuji Sagara[1], Bungo Furusato[2], Junya Fukuoka[2], Hideki Sakai[1]

[1]Department of Urology, Nagasaki University Graduate School of Biomedical Sciences, Nagasaki, Japan, [2]Department of Pathology, Nagasaki University Graduate School of Biomedical Sciences, Nagasaki, Japan

Keywords: human antigen R, angiogenesis, lymphangiogenesis, vascular endothelial growth factor, bladder cancer

Background: Green tea is known to have health-promoting effects that are attributed to catechin polyphenols, which have anti-inflammatory and -oxidative properties. Many studies have demonstrated the anti-cancer effects of green tea polyphenol (GTP) in a variety of malignancies including bladder cancer, and epidemiologic studies have shown that green tea consumption reduces cancer risk. New cancer treatment strategies in combination with GTP intake have been recommended for several types of cancer. Thus, GTP is thought to be useful not only for cancer prevention, but also for treatment. However, the mechanistic basis of these effects is not well understood.

Objective: To clarify the molecular mechanisms of GTP-induced anti-cancer effects, we used a mouse model of chemically induced bladder cancer.

Methods: C3H/He mice (8 weeks old; n = 46) were treated with 0.05% N-butyl-N- (4-hydroxybutyl) nitrosamine (BBN) solution for 14–24 weeks. Mice in the BBN + GTP group (n = 47) were also treated with 0.5% GTP solution over the same period. Tumor cell proliferation, and microvessel density were evaluated along with immunohistochemical analysis of human antigen R (HuR), vascular endothelial growth factor (VEGF)-A, cyclooxygenase (COX)-2, and hemeoxygenase (HO)-1 expression.

Results: Cytoplasmic HuR expression in cancer cells was higher at 14 and 24 weeks in the BBN than in the control group and was associated with increased invasion of tumor cells in muscle. However, these effects were not observed in the BBN + GTP group. A multivariate analysis of GTP intake and cytoplasmic HuR expression revealed that GTP was independently associated with COX-2 and HO-1 expression, while cytoplasmic HuR expression was associated with COX-2 and VEGF-A levels. Expression of COX-2 and HO-1 was associated with cell proliferation and that of VEGF-A and HO-1 was associated with angiogenesis. In regard to nuclear HuR, its expression was not associated with any parameters, such as carcinogenesis, muscle invasion, and GTP intake.

Conclusion: Our results supported the opinion that GTP intake can suppress tumor progression and malignant behavior in animal model of bladder cancer. In addition, we speculate that GTP directly and indirectly suppresses tumor cell proliferation and angiogenesis via HuR-related pathways in bladder cancer tissue.

INHIBITORY EFFECT OF CITRUS PEEL ON COLON CARCINOGENESIS WITH SUPPRESSION OF OXIDATIVE STRESS

Keiji Wakabayashi[1], Susumu Tomono[1], and Michihiro Mutoh[2]

[1]Graduate Division of Nutritional and Environmental Sciences, University of Shizuoka, Shizuoka, Japan; [2]Epidemiology and Prevention Group, Research Center for Cancer Prevention and Screening, National Cancer Center, Tokyo, Japan

Keywords: citrus peel, oxidative stress, Nrf2, aberrant crypt foci, colon carcinogenesis

Background: Oxidative stress status generated by reactive oxygen species (ROS) modifies DNA bases that induce DNA damage, and it also induces lipid peroxidation, both of which are likely to play an important role in carcinogenesis. In addition, ROS proliferate cancer cells and block apoptosis of cancer cells through activation of activator protein-1 (AP-1) and nuclear factor-kappaB (NF-κB) transcription factors. Previous studies demonstrated that orange extracts show strong antioxidant potential *in vitro and in vivo* experiments, and oral administration of citrus peel extracts has wound healing effects on the skin of diabetic rats. Recently, we reported that oral administration of limonoids present in citrus fruits inhibits intestinal tumorigenesis in *Apc*-mutant Min mice.

Objective: Since dietary citrus has been shown to reduce oxidative stress, in this study, we investigated the effects of dried citrus peel on the activity of oxidative stress-related transcriptional factors in cultured cancer cell line, and colon carcinogenesis in rats.

Methods: The effects of citrus (*Citrus tangerina*) peel extract containing flavonoids and carotenoids on the activity of oxidative stress-related transcriptional factors, including AP-1, NF-κB, NRF2, p53 and STAT3, were investigated in human colon cancer cell line, Caco-2 cells, using a luciferase reporter gene assay. For the induction of aberrant crypt foci (ACF) by azoxymethane (AOM), 6-week-old male F344 rats were given intraperitoneal injections of AOM (15 mg/kg-body) for twice at one week. A day after the last AOM injection, the rats were fed with AIN-76A diet containing 0 and 1000 ppm ground citrus peel for 4 weeks. At the end of the experimental period, the colorectum was removed, opened longitudinally and fixed flat between sheets of filter paper in 10% buffered formalin for more than 24 hr. They were divided into the proximal segment, rectum (1.5 cm in length), then the proximal (middle) and distal halves of the remainder. These were stained with 0.2% methylene blue and the mucosal surface was assessed for ACF with a stereoscopic microscope.

Results: AP-1, NF-κB, NRF2, p53 and STAT3 transcriptional activities were tested with diluted ethanol extracts of dried citrus peel, and NRF2 transcriptional activities were found to increase 2.0-fold of the untreated control value at dilution of 1/2000. On the other hand, NF-κB, p53 and STAT3 transcriptional activities were slightly decreased compared to the untreated control value. All F344 rats treated with AOM developed ACF in the colorectum. There is no difference in body weight and food intake between control and citrus peel group. The total numbers of ACF in the group treated with citrus peel at 1000 ppm were reduced to 75 % ($p<0.01$) of the control value. The number of focus consisting of 2ACs were also decreased.

Conclusion: These results indicate that citrus peel might block cellular oxidative stress through induction of NRF2, and prevent colon carcinogenesis.

PROTECTIVE INFLUENCE OF VIRGIN COCONUT *COCOS NUCIFERA* OIL SUPPLEMENTATION AGAINST THE DEVELOPMENT OF N-METHYL-N-NITROSOUREA-INDUCED MAMMARY NEOPLASIA IN A MURINE MODEL

M.L.C. Mann[1], P.E.E. Calderon[1,2], J. F. Domingo[1], C.M.C. Torralba[1], V.M.F.V. Banal[1], H.S.A. Lastrilla[1], M.L. Cavaneyro[1], A.C. Valenciano[1], J.C.D. Vicente[1], K.B. Villano[1], E.I.B.S. Lintag[1], A.C.M. Aguinaldo[1], K.N.M. Manalastas[1], K.M. Labriaga[1], R.F.P. Miranda[1], and E.J.E. Calderon[3]

[1]College of Medicine, San Beda College, 638 Mendiola Street, San Miguel, Manila, Philippines; [2]Biology Department, College of Science, De La Salle University, 2401 Taft Avenue, Manila, Philippines; [3]College of Medicine, Pamantasan ng Lungsod ng Maynila (University of the City of Manila), Intramuros, Manila, Philippines

Keywords: mammary neoplasia, breast cancer, N-methyl-N-nitrosourea, *Cocos nucifera*, virgin coconut oil

Background: Breast cancer is the most frequently diagnosed life-threatening cancer in women in the world. In developing countries such as the Philippines, it is the leading cause of cancer death among women. To date, it is projected that 3/100 Filipino women will develop breast cancer before age 75 and 1/100 will die before reaching 75. Over the past three decades, extensive breast cancer research has led to extraordinary progress in the understanding of the disease, resulting in the development of more targeted treatments and preventive strategies. Interestingly, emerging epidemiological and experimental evidences suggest a relationship between dietary fat intake and the risk of cancer. Modern research has demonstrated a number of potential benefits of virgin coconut

Cocos nucifera (Arecales: Arecaceae) oil on health. VCO is easily extracted from the kernel or meat of the mature coconut and is widely available in Southeast Asia. In an effort to explore the benefits of functional food for possibly reducing cancer-related morbidity and mortality, this study was conducted as a pilot investigation on the potential protective influence of VCO supplementation against the development of experimental mammary neoplasia in an animal model.

Objectives: The objective of this study was to evaluate the effects of oral supplementation with VCO for 60 days on the development of mammary neoplasia in adult virgin female Sprague-Dawley rats treated with N-methyl-N-nitrosourea (NMU). Specifically, the histological incidence and histopathological features of the mammary neoplasia that developed were determined.

Methods: Thirty (30) two-week old virgin female Sprague-Dawley rats were randomly assigned to six treatment groups: (1) sham (plain normal saline solution [PNSS] only), (2) NMU control, (3) VCO5 control (VCO 5 mL/kg body weight), (4) VCO10 control (VCO 10 mL/kg body weight), (5) VCO5 + NMU, and (6) VCO10 + NMU. Standard laboratory-grade VCO procured from the Philippines was used in this study. Oral supplementation with VCO was done daily for 60 days via gastric gavage. To induce mammary neoplasia, a single dose of NMU 50mg/kg was given intraperitoneally to the NMU control and to the experimental groups VCO5 + NMU and VCO10 + NMU on the 15th day of VCO treatment. There was no mortality among the subjects during and after the administration of NMU. One day after the last dose of VCO supplementation, surgical harvest of mammary tissue was done under pentobarbital anesthesia. The mammary tissues were excised, washed with saline solution, and placed in 10% buffered formalin solution. Paraffin sections (5 μm thick) were prepared from each mammary gland and were stained with hematoxylin and eosin. The tissues were examined under light microscopy. The histological incidence and histopathological features of the mammary neoplasia that developed were determined.

Results: There was no mortality among the subjects during the 60-day study period. The mammary tissues from the sham, VCO 5, VCO 10, and VCO 10 + NMU groups were normal and were negative for neoplasia. Pre-malignant neoplasms were noted in the NMU control (60%) and VCO 5 + NMU (40%) groups. There was a significant reduction in the incidence of mammary neoplasia in the mammary tissues of the VCO-treated groups ($p < 0.05$). The pre-malignant changes noted included epithelial and ductal hyperplasia. Hyperchromatic and large nucleus with some pleomorphism were likewise noted. No malignant features were observed.

Conclusion: Oral supplementation with VCO for 60 days significantly attenuated the development of mammary neoplasia in adult virgin female Sprague-Dawley rats treated with N-methyl-N-nitrosourea.

WHAT'S IN YOUR DIETARY FIBER SUPPLEMENT? USING THE DIETARY SUPPLEMENT LABEL DATABASE (DSLD) TO DETERMINE TOTAL DIETARY FIBER LEVELS FOR USE IN ONCOLOGY COMMUNITY HEALTH CARE.

Nancy J. Emenaker[1], Barbara C. Sorkin[2], Johanna T. Dwyer[2], Luz M. Rodriguez[3,4]

[1]NSRG, NCI, NIH, Bethesda, MD, USA; [2]ODS, NIH, OD, Bethesda, MD, USA; [3]GOCRG, NCI, NIH, Bethesda, MD, USA; [4]Walter Reed National Military Medical Center, Dept. of Surgery, Bethesda, MD, USA

Keywords: dietary supplements, dietary fiber, colon health, colon cancer, supplement facts panel, community health care

Background: More than 50% of all U.S. adults consume dietary supplements (DS) to promote health and well-being contributing to an estimated $35 billion in sales in 2015. An estimated 26-77% of cancer patients and long-term survivors report using any type of DS after diagnosis. Dietary fiber containing supplements are often recommended by the oncology community (e.g., oncology health care professionals, researchers and patients) to promote bowel health and reduce disease risks, including risk of colorectal cancer. Yet, DS can contribute greatly to total nutrient intake and may go underreported in clinical care. DS product entry and exit from the U.S. marketplace, combined with product variations and reformulations, may pose considerable issues for health care providers and others when determining total overall intakes in individuals using some DS products.

Objective: We examined the NIH dietary supplement label database (DSLD), a web-based interface; containing over 50,000

U.S. commercially available DS products to determine amounts and types of dietary fiber in these products per manufacturer's supplement label panels.

Methods: We searched DSLD for all products including the terms "fiber", "dietary fiber", "soluble fiber", "insoluble fiber", "colon cleanse" and "colon health" as either a product name, dietary ingredient, brand name, or label element hypothesized to affect cancer outcomes.

Results: DSLD yielded a total of 4,873 products containing the search term "fiber" anywhere on the product label. A total of 181 products contained ingredients classified as "fiber" and 196 products contained "fiber" in the product name. 3,526 products contained "dietary fiber" anywhere on the label and 5 contained "dietary fiber" in the dietary ingredient name. 480 contained "soluble fiber" anywhere on the label. Of the 6 products that contained "soluble fiber" in the product name, only 3 products contained "soluble fiber" in the ingredient name. Similarly, of the 201 products that contained "insoluble fiber" anywhere on the label, 1 product contained "insoluble fiber" as a dietary ingredient name. 109 products contained "colon cleanse" anywhere on the product label; 58 contained "colon cleanse" on in the product name; and one contained "colon cleanse" in the dietary ingredient name. Finally, 235 products contained "colon health" anywhere on the label, and 5 contained "colon health" in the product name. DSLD can also be used in some cases to determine the type(s) of fiber claimed as present in each product, providing the potential for assessment of intake of fiber intake and may assist the oncology community in differentiating fiber intake into soluble vs insoluble fiber categories for assessing total fiber intake.

Conclusion: DSLD serves as an online resource supplying a broad range of users, including oncology practitioners with relevant DS information for research and clinical use. Funding: Office of Dietary Supplements and the National Library of Medicine, National Institutes of Health.

THE IMMUNO-MODULATORY AND ANTI-PROLIFERATIVE ACTIVITY OF HIGH MOLECULAR WEIGHT AND MODIFIED CITRUS PECTIN

Rihab Al-Merheb, Venicia Hawach, Marc Karam, Roula M. Abdel-Massih

Department of Biology, University of Balamand, Al-Koura, Lebanon

Keywords: Immuno-modulatory, anti-proliferative, pectin

Background: Pectin is a heterogeneous polysaccharide mainly present in citrus fruits and has different biological activities.

Objective: High molecular weight Citrus Pectin and modified citrus pectin (MCP) were tested for their immunomodulatory, cytotoxic, and anti-proliferative activity.

Methods: Twenty-eight BALB/c mice were fed *ad libitum* different concentrations (1.5%, 3%, and 5%) of pectin or MCP on a daily basis for three weeks. ELISA Development Kits were used to test the immunomodulatory activity of different pectins and MCPs. The cytotoxicity of pectin was studied against HaCaT cell line using Trypan blue method and a non-radioactive LDH-cytotoxicity assay. Anti-proliferative activity was assayed using a WST-1 proliferation kit.

Results: Pectin and MCP induced TNFα, IFN γ, IL1β, IL-4, IL-10 and IL-17 cytokines production at different levels. Cytotoxicity of various concentrations of pectin and MCP was studied against HaCaT cell line and IC$_{50}$ was calculated. MCP was found to be more cytotoxic than high molecular weight citrus pectin since it had a lower IC$_{50}$ (300ug/ul). At non-cytotoxic concentrations, the viability of cells decreased with increase of concentration of MCP as determined by the WST-1. Biological activity of pectin varied according to the source of the pectin extract and the molecular weight of pectin

Conclusion: The conclusions from this study suggest that MCP exhibit a higher anti-proliferative effect on HaCaT cell line than pectin. The immunomodulatory effect is still under investigation.

PROTECTIVE EFFECTS OF SULFORAPHANE ON HUMAN BLADDER CANCER BOTH *IN VIVO* AND *IN VITRO*

Yujuan Shan[1,2*], Lei Huang[1], Peng Lei[1], Xiaodong Liu[1]

[1]School of Chemistry and Chemical Engineering, Harbin Institute of Technology, Harbin, 150090, China; [2]MIIT Key Laboratory of Critical Materials Technology for New Energy Conversion and Storage, School of Chemistry and Chemical Engineering, Harbin Institute of Technology

Keywords: sulforaphane, bladder cancer, signal pathway

Background: Sulforaphane is one of the isothiocyanates (ITCs), which are abundantly and exclusively existed as precursors of glucosinolates (GS) in quite a few of cruciferous vegetables, especially in broccoli sprout. Although at least 120 different GS have been identified, only a small number of ITCs such as sulforaphane, allyl-isothiocyanate, Benzyl-isothiocyanate, and Phenethyl-isothiocyanate, may be commonly consumed by humans. Generally, ITCs ingested orally are metabolized principally by the mercapturic acid pathway. They are experienced to a series of enzymatic conjugation and ultimately metabolized to NAC (N-Acetyl-Cys) ITC, which presents the similar functions as their parental compounds. Sulforaphane has been proved to have effective anti-cancer property, while the potential inhibition mechanism is still not very perfect. In this study, some specific targets and signaling pathways involved in the inhibition of bladder cancer were studied in vitro and in vivo.

Objectives: The aim of the present study was to investigate the protective effect of sulforaphane on bladder cancer.

Methods: The male athymic mice were injected subcutaneously with UM-UC-3 cell for xenograft assay. The histopathologic differences of tumor tissues were stained with histologic examination. Microarray Arrays was used to analyze the changes in miRNA expression. The miR-200c mimic and inhibitor was transfected into T24 cells, and miR-200c expression was analyzed by real-time PCR. The overexpression and gene silencing effects of COX-2 and MMP-2/-9 were performed with overexpression plasmids and small-interference RNA, separately. The protein expression of phase 2 detoxification enzymes and COX-2/MMP-2/MMP-9 were analyzed by western blotting. The cell cycle arrest and apoptosis were analyzed by flow cytometry. In addition, the effect of sulforaphane on T24 cell metastasis and invasion were analyzed by scratch wound and inverted invasion assays, respectively.

Results: In vivo, sulforaphane reduced tumor cell angiogenesis, significantly decreased the volume and size of UM-UC-3 xenograft tumor and the areas of necrosis in nu/nu mice. In human bladder cancer T24 cells, sulforaphane inhibited the epithelial-to-mesenchymal transition process and suppressed tumor cell invasion and migration by two different pathways: 1) Sulforaphane activated p38 MAPK then inhibited NF- k B binding to the COX-2 promoter, thereby inhibited the expression of COX-2 and its downstream MMP-2/-9 and Snail/ZEB1; 2) After treated with sulforaphane for 24 h, twelve genes miRNA were up-regulated more than 2 times and fifteen genes miRNA were down-regulated significantly. Importantly, sulforaphane up-regulated miR200c expression and inhibited its downstream transcriptional factor (ZEB1). Ultimately, sulforaphane induced E-cadherin expression by the two pathways and followed by the inhibitory effect on epithelial-to-mesenchymal transition and metastasis. Moreover, sulforaphane activated p38 MAPK and then promoted the translocation of Nrf-2 into nucleus, which followed with induction of phase 2 detoxification enzymes (NQO1, TrxR-1, and GST1A1). Besides, sulforaphane induced the early apoptosis and cell cycle arrest at G_1/S phase through up-regulating p27, an inhibitor of cyclin-dependent kinase.

Conclusion: The present results indicated that sulforaphane, naturally existing in cruciferous vegetables, could be a potential and beneficial agent for human bladder cancer.

THE EFFECT OF KEFIR PRODUCED FROM THE NATURAL KEFIR GRAINS ON THE INTESTINAL MICROORGANISMS OF THE BALB/C MICE

Fatih Selim Erdoğan, Seda Kurtulmus, Tugba Kok Tas, Zeynep B. Guzel Seydim

Suleyman Demirel University Faculty of Engineering Department of Food Engineering, Isparta 32260 Turkey

Keywords: kefir, kefir grains, probiotic, intestinal microorganism, mold, *Trichoderma koningii*

Background: Kefir is a probiotic and fermented dairy product, which is authentically produced from kefir grains. Kefir grains contain numerous lactic acid bacteria and yeasts within a polysaccharide structure. Kefir is a miraculous food regarding its favorable contributions to the human health. It has beneficial effects on the immunity and digestive/gastrointestinal system in addition to its cholesterol-lowering, lactose intolerance preventing, antimutagenic, anticarcinogenic and antimicrobial properties. However, kefir starter cultures used in industrial kefir productions contains very few lactic acid bacteria and don't contain yeasts.

Objective: The objective of this study was to compare the intestinal microorganisms of the BALB/c mice fed with kefir produced from natural kefir grains and from the industrial starter culture.

Methods: Kefir samples were produced from the kefir grains and kefir starter culture. The lactic acid bacteria (LAB) content of kefir samples produced from the kefir grains and the starter culture were 10.53 log CFU/ml and 8.42 log CFU/ml respectively, and yeast contents were 6.94 log CFU/ml and 2.25 log CFU/ml, respectively. BALB/c mice were divided into three groups as control group, grain group and starter culture group. The mice were fed with an oral dose of 0.3µl/day for 15 days, and their feces were collected in metabolic cages (Days 0, 3, 5, 7, 9, 11, 13 and 15). The lactic acid bacteria, yeasts-fungi, *L. acidophilus and Bifidobacterium* species were determined. Additionally, PCR analysis based on yeast-fungus 23S-rRNA was carried out, and the serial analysis was determined with ABI 3100 Genetic Analyzer.

Results: The mean LAB contents of the feces samples obtained from the mice, which were fed 15 days long with the kefir samples produced from the kefir grains and starter culture, were 9.08 log CFU/ml; 7.32 log CFU/ml respectively. After the 7th day, there was a significant difference in respect of lactic acid bacteria contents due to the effects of t in the stool of the mice fed with authentic kefir produced from the kefir grains was 4.58 log CFU/ml on the first day, no yeast proliferation was observed in the mice fed with the kefir produced from the starter culture. It was noted that fungus content was 5.09 log CFU/ml in both starter kefir group and in the control group. It was very impressive that unlike from other groups, no fungus colonies were observed in the feces samples of the mice fed with the kefir produced from kefir grains. The fungus was identified as *Trichoderma koningii* that is a potential human pathogen and cancerogen.

Conclusion: There are several studies focused on the antimicrobial effects of kefir. This study might lead to new studies focused on the antifungal effects of kefir.

EFFECT OF KEFIR ON *FUSOBACTERIUM NUCLEATUM* POTENTIALLY CAUSING INTESTINAL CANCER

Zeynep Banu Güzel-Seydim, Merve Dibekçi, Ece Çağdaş, Atıf Can Seydim

Suleyman Demirel University Faculty of Engineering Department of Food Engineering Isparta 32260 Turkey

Keywords: *Fuscobacterium nucleatum*, pathogen, carcinogen, fermented foods, kefir, kefir grains

Background: *Fusobacterium* spp. are known to be part of the mouth and intestinal microbiota. *Fusobacterium nucleatum* is an obligate anaerobe, gram negative, non-spore former, and pleomorphic bacillus that can cause diseases mainly not only in the mouth and teeth also in brain, pleura, lungs and liver. It was also noted that *F. nucleatum* induces fetal death (fetal demise) in pregnant women. Recent studies implicate that *F. nucleatum* could lead to colon cancer by binding the epithelial tissue. Kefir is originally produced from kefir grains that are actually a mine of probiotics. Fermented dairy products especially kefir and yogurt are significant for functional nutrition. Lactic acid bacteria, acetic acid bacteria and yeasts are embedded in a polysaccharide matrix, called kefiran, in kefir grains. When kefir grains are added to milk and incubated for approximately 22 h at 25°C, microorganisms in the grains continue to proliferate in milk with the production of the functional metabolic compounds. While yogurt has mainly two bacteria, authentic kefir has its characteristic *Lactobacillus kefiranofaciens*, *Lactobacillus kefir* and *Lactobacillus parakefir* in addition to many other types of LAB. Previous studies have indicated that fermented dairy products can cause probiotic effects such as improvement in digestive system health, serum cholesterol reduction, and improvement in lactose tolerance, improved immune function, control of irritable bowel symptoms, as well as anticarcinogenic properties.

Objective: The aim of this research is to report the effects of fermented dairy products *in vitro* growth of *F. nucleatum. Milk,* kefir made from natural kefir grains, industrial kefir produced from kefir starter culture, yogurt produced from natural yogurt starter culture and industrial yogurt produced from yogurt starter culture were used against *F. nucleatum.*

Methods: *F. nucleatum* (ATCC 25586) was grown in Fluid Thioglicollate Medium at 37°C for 3 days under anaerobic incubation. Kefir was made from authentic kefir grains with 2% inoculation at 25°C for 22h fermentation. Yogurt was made with using a natural starter culture. Inhibition effect of fermented dairy products was determined *in vitro* against to *F. nucleatum.* Kirby Bauer Method was used for zone inhibition test; sterile disks that were dunk into kefir and yogurt samples were placed on Brucella Blood Agar with Hemin and Vitamin K1 inoculated with *F. nucleatum* and incubated at 37°C for 3 days under anaerobic conditions. Inhibition zones were determined after incubation completion. In addition, both lactic acid bacteria (counted on MRS and m17), yeast (PDA) and related pathogen were observed after anaerobic incubation by adding a certain amount of kefir and yogurt cultures into *F. nucleatum* inoculated medium.

Results: Authentic kefir samples exhibited distinct inhibitory zone against *F. nucleatum* after incubation agar plates. The largest zone of inhibition (with 9.42 mm) was determined in natural kefir sample made from kefir grains. Yogurt sample provided 8.25mm zone inhibition against *F. nucleatum.* Milk used in kefir and yogurt making did not form any zone of inhibition. It was also found that number of *F. nucleatum* in Thioglicollate Medium decreased depending on inoculated concentrations of kefir and yogurt cultures.

Conclusion: Kefir is known to have positive effects on health, especially intestinal health; therefore, these findings are important since inhibition effect of fermented dairy products against a pathogen and possible carcinogen was shown. Regular consumption of natural fermented dairy products especially kefir should be included in a functional diet. It could be promising to investigate with *in vivo* studies.

Part 8
Prebiotics, Probiotics, and Cancer

WATER BUFFALO MOZZARELLA CHEESE AS A SOURCE OF POTENTIAL PROBIOTIC LACTIC ACID BACTERIA FOR APPLICATION IN FUNCTIONAL FOOD

Liane Caroline Sousa Nascimento[1], Sabrina Neves Casarotti[1], Luana Faria Silva[1] and Ana Lúcia Barretto Penna[1]

[1]UNESP, São Paulo State University, Department of Food Engineering and Technology, São José do Rio Preto, SP, Brazil

Keywords: *Enterococcus* spp., gastrointestinal conditions, safety, technological properties

Background: *Enterococcus* spp. and *Lactobacillus* spp. have shown several probiotic characteristics, which are valuable for the development of novel functional products with technological profile for commercial purpose and therapeutic properties among the consumers.

Objective: To evaluate the technological profile, probiotic potential and safety of lactic acid bacteria strains, previously isolated from water buffalo mozzarella cheese.

Methods: A preliminary screening using twenty-one strains of lactic acid bacteria (LAB), belonging to Enterococci and Lactobacilli genera was carried out by means of the technological properties (acidification profile, viability in different temperatures, pH values, NaCl and bile salts concentration, proteolytic activity, ability to use citrate and production of CO_2, organic acids, acetoin and diacetyl), probiotic potential (bile salts hydrolase - BSH activity, auto-aggregation, co-aggregation and hydrophobicity), and safety (susceptibility to antibiotics, mucin degradation, and presence of virulence factors). Taking all the results into account, strains with better probiotic potential were submitted to additional tests of production of ®-galactosidase, survival to simulated gastrointestinal (GI) conditions and adhesion to Caco-2 cells.

Results: Most of the strains grew well at 30 °C, was viable in the presence of 6.5% NaCl and 3% bile salts, produced protease, reduced the pH to ≤ 5.0, and produced high concentration of organic compounds. *Enterococcus* sp. strains were characterized by their production of acetic, formic, and pyruvic acids, and *Lb. helveticus* and *Lb. delbrueckii* subsp. *bulgaricus* were characterized by their production of acetoin, while the production of lactic acid was related to *Lb. delbrueckii* subsp. *bulgaricus.* Six strains presented BSH activity and most of them presented high value of auto-aggregation and hydrophobicity. Some strains presented co-aggregation capacity with other LAB and pathogens. None of the strains degraded the mucin; however, all of them presented resistance to vancomycin and kanamycin and 95% of them were resistant to gentamycin. The strains *Enterococcus faecium* SJRP20 and SJRP65 were selected considering their technological and probiotic features, and safety. Both strains resisted well to the GIT stress conditions (> 8 log CFU/mL), presented low adherence to Caco-2 cells (5.7-8.4%), and are β-galactosidase enzyme producers.

Conclusion: The strains *Enterococcus faecium* SJRP20 and SJRP65 presented good technological and functional properties, with interesting features for application in food products. Further *in vivo* tests must be carried out to guarantee their safety and probiotic potential prior to their application in functional food.

SELECTION OF *LACTOBACILLUS* SPP. STRAINS FOR THE DEVELOPMENT OF INNOVATIVE PROBIOTIC FUNCTIONAL FERMENTED PRODUCTS

Bruna Maria Salotti de Souza[1], Luana Faria Silva[1], Sabrina Neves Casarotti[1] and Ana Lúcia Barretto Penna[1]

[1]UNESP, São Paulo State University, Department of Food Engineering and Technology, São José do Rio Preto, SP, Brazil

Keywords: lactic acid bacteria, fermented milk, simulation of gastrointestinal conditions, technological properties.

Background: The consumption of probiotic products results in the balance of the intestinal microbiota, which has a favorable impact on consumer health. The proper selection of strains should be carefully conducted to guarantee their safety, and technological and probiotic properties for commercial purposes.

Objective: To investigate the technological and probiotic potential of lactic acid bacteria (LAB) strains, and to select novel strains to be applied in innovative functional fermented products.

Methods: Thirteen *Lactobacillus casei* and seven *Lactobacillus fermentum* strains isolated from mozzarella cheese were technologically characterized by the acidification profile, viability in different temperatures, pH values and NaCl concentrations, proteolytic activity, ability to use citrate and production of CO_2, organic acids, acetoin and diacetyl (Silva, 2010). The probiotic potential was evaluated by the susceptibility to antibiotics by the agar disc diffusion test (Charteris et al., 1998), auto-aggregation and co-aggregation (Todorov et al., 2011), cell surface hydrophobicity (Todorov and Dicks, 2008), production of β-galactosidase (Vinderola and Reinheimer, 2003) and tolerance to simulated gastrointestinal (GI) tract conditions (Bautista-Gallego et al. 2013).

Results: *Lb. fermentum* strains grew at 45 °C, while *Lb. casei* showed growth at different temperatures; the optimal growth was observed between 12-18 h. *Lb. fermentum* and most of *Lb. casei* are positive-citrate, produced protease, and most of the strains reduced the milk pH value to 5.0 after 18 h of fermentation, being considered slow in dairy fermentation. Strains of *Lb. fermentum* produced CO_2 from glucose. *Lb. casei* strains were characterized by the production of lactic acid while the production of acetic, formic and pyruvic acids was a feature of *Lb. fermentum*. All strains were resistant to vancomycin and the vast majority (65%) of strains were resistant to kanamycin. Almost all strains of both species showed high auto-aggregation, and some strains showed co-aggregation ability with other LAB and/or pathogens, and *Lb. casei* SJRP48 and *Lb. fermentum* SJRP32 demonstrated the highest co-aggregation values (72-96%). In general, both species showed wide range of hydrophobicity values, although *Lb. casei* SPRP39 and *Lb. fermentum* SJRP164 differed (>60%) from the others. Most of *Lb. casei* strains and all strains of *Lb. fermentum* produced β-galactosidase enzyme, except for SJRP60. The strains of *Lb. casei* SJRP38, SJRP147 and SJRP166 and *Lb. fermentum* SJRP46, SJRP60 and SJRP164 survived well (> 6 log CFU/mL) the simulation of stressful conditions of the gastrointestinal tract.

Conclusion: Considering the overall results, the strains of *Lactobacillus casei* SJRP38 and *Lactobacillus fermentum* SJRP43 presented good technological features and high probiotic potential for further application in functional fermented products.

POTENTIAL BENEFITS OF PROBIOTICS CONSUMPTION

Gabriela Riscuta

Nutritional Science Research Group, Division of Cancer Prevention, National Cancer Institute, Bethesda MD, USA

Marketing and consumption of probiotic products is growing exponentially, despite the gap in knowledge regarding their safety and efficacy. Nevertheless, some probiotics have shown benefits in specific conditions. A number of probiotics administered alone or in combination, as capsules or added to fermented dairies, were able to partially improve symptoms related to irritable bowel syndrome, diarrhea caused by antibiotics or chemotherapy, periodontitis, etc. Since probiotics were administered in different dosages and combinations, expectedly, showed different results, more or less significant. Usually, the magnitude of the effect depends by the type, dose, and combination of probiotics administered and by the severity and the type of the condition for which were administered. More research is needed to better understand the effects of probiotics, singly, or in combination, and the actions of microbial metabolites on the host in the context of complex interactions with food, dietary patterns, antibiotics and other prescribed medications, health status, gender, age, etc. There is a need to accelerate the research for substantiating measurable functional benefits of probiotic/prebiotic components and/or their combination and to understand the underlying mechanisms of their action(s), along with the variability in responses to these interventions.

EFFECTS OF *L. PARACASEI* SUBP. *PARACASEI* X12 ON CELL CYCLE OF COLON CANCER HT-29 CELLS AND REGULATION OF MTOR SIGNALING PATHWAY

Lei Huang[1], Kaikai Li[1], Peng Lei[1], Xiaodong Liu[1], and Yujuan Shan[1]

[1] School of Chemistry and Chemical Engineering, Harbin Institute of Technology, Harbin, 150090, China

Keywords: probiotics, colon cancer, cell cycle, mTOR signaling pathway

Background: Colon cancer has become a common malignant tumour occurring in the digestive tract. At present, the drugs used for chemotherapy still have some unwished curative effects. Probiotics such as *Lactobacillus* spp. are proven to have effective anti-cancer function and no side effect, while the potential inhibition mechanism is still not very perfect. In this study, *L. paracasei* subp. *paracasei* X12 is newly separated from the traditional cheese in Xinjiang Province (China) by our group. Through previous screening experiments, *L. paracasei* subp. *paracasei* X12 exhibits the distinctive inhibition of proliferation in human colon cancer HT-29 cells and has great potential for further application.

Objective: The research is aimed at finding key targets and the impact of *L. paracasei* subp. *paracasei* X12 on colon cancer HT-29, providing a theoretical basis for the further development and application of *Lactobacillus*.

Methods: Flow cytometry (PI single staining method) was used to detect the effects of *L. paracasei* subp. *paracasei* X12 on colon cancer cell cycle with different multiplicity of infection (MOI 0,

10, 50, 100) for 24 h and 48 h. Then in order to determine the specific regulators involved, cyclin E_1 and cyclin D_1, the positive regulators, and p16, p27, the negative regulatory factors were further explored by RT-PCR technique. Finally, to further understand whether mTOR signaling takes the crucial roles in *Lactobacillus* X12-mediated cell cycle arrest, HT-29 cells were transiently transfected with plasmid of $p^{cDNA3-1mTOR}$.

Results: After treatment with *Lactobacillus* X12 at different MOI (0, 10, 50 and 100) for 24 h, the percentage of cells at G_1 phase was increased in a dose-dependent manner. The expressions of cyclin E_1 mRNA were significantly decreased by 31, 33 and 59% at 24 h and 29, 77 and 75% at 48 h after incubation with different doses of *Lactobacillus* X12, and significant reduction of cyclin D_1 mRNA was observed at 48 h. In sharp contrast, p27 mRNA expressions but not p16 were increased to 1.6 folds, 1.8 folds, 2.1 folds at 24 h treatment point and to 2.8 folds, 3.1 folds, 3.9 folds at 48 h treatment point. The level of mTOR gene expression was greatly suppressed by 42-48% after treatment with *Lactobacillus* X12 for 24 h. $4EBP_1$ mRNA was obviously induced to 1.8-2.4 folds, while there is no significant effect on p70S6K. Furthermore, *Lactobacillus* X12 (MOI 50) can remarkably reverse the decreased levels of p27 mRNA which is controlled by plasmid of $p^{cDNA3-1mTOR}$. Unlike p27, cyclin E_1 mRNA was not obviously changed with mTOR.

Conclusion: The present findings suggested that *L. paracasei* subp. *paracasei* X12 can block colon cancer HT-29 cell cycle at G_1 checkpoint through inhibiting cyclin E_1 and cyclin D_1, meanwhile enhancing p27, which were mediated by $mTOR/4EBP_1$ signaling pathway. These results will provide a theoretical basis for further development of *Lactobacillus*.

LACTOBACILLUS GASSERI SBT2055 STIMULATES IMMUNOGLOBULIN PRODUCTION AND INNATE IMMUNITY AFTER INFLUENZA VACCINATION IN HEALTHY ADULT VOLUNTEERS: A RANDOMIZED, DOUBLE-BLIND, PLACEBO-CONTROLLED, PARALLEL-GROUP STUDY

Jun Nishihira[1], Tomohiro Moriya[2], Fumihiko Sakai[2], Toshihide Kabuki[2], Yoshihiro Kawasaki[2], and Mie Nishimura[1]

[1]Health Information Science Center, Hokkaido Information University, Ebetsu, Hokkaido 069-8585, Japan; [2]Milk Science Research Institute, Megmilk Snow Brand Co. Ltd., Minamidai, Kawagoe, Saitama 350-1165, Japan

Keywords: clinical trial, influenza vaccine, lactobacillus gasseri, natural killer cell

Background: *Lactobacillus gasseri* strain SBT2055 (LG2055) is a human intestine-originating probiotic bacterium and potent probiotic known to exert various health promotion effects, including prevention of abdominal adiposity in rats and humans. A recent finding in mice has suggested that oral administration of LG2055 induces a protective effect against influenza A virus infection. To confirm this in humans, a human clinical trial was performed.

Methods: A randomized, double-blind, placebo-controlled, parallel-group study in healthy adult volunteers was conducted to examine the effect of drinkable yogurt (DY) containing LG2055 on influenza vaccine-specific antibody responses as the primary objective and innate immune responses as the secondary objective. Subjects were asked to consume 100 g/day of DY with LG2055 (LG2055 group; n = 94) or without LG2055 (placebo group; n =

94) for 16 weeks. After 4 weeks, all subjects received a trivalent influenza vaccine.

Results: We found that the intake of LG2055 DY increased hemagglutination inhibition titers against influenza viruses A/H1N1 and B and the rate of seroprotection against influenza B after vaccination as compared with the intake of placebo DY by healthy volunteers. In support of this result. we confirmed that total IgG and IgA levels in plasma and sIgA production in saliva were also higher in the LG2055 group than in the placebo group. Furthermore, the intake of LG2055 DY enhanced natural killer cell activity and myxovirus resistance A gene expression, which is one of the antiviral genes stimulated by type I or type III Interferons in peripheral blood mononuclear cells.

Conclusion: The results obtained in this study strongly indicate that LG2055 activates both the innate and adaptive human immune responses, suggesting the potential to prevent influenza virus infections by providing specific probiotics as complementary foods.

Part 9
Prevention and Management of Dementia

THE ROLE OF LUTEIN IN COGNITIVE FUNCTION: A REVIEW

E.J. Johnson

Jean Mayer USDA Human Nutrition Research Center on Aging at Tufts University, Boston, MA, USA

Keywords: lutein, macular pigment, cognition, aging

Epidemiological studies suggest that dietary lutein may be of benefit in maintaining cognitive health. Among the carotenoids, lutein and its isomer zeaxanthin, are the only two that cross the blood-retina barrier to form macular pigment (MP) in the eye. Lutein also preferentially accumulates in human brain. Lutein and zeaxanthin in macula were found to be significantly correlated with their levels in matched brain tissue. Therefore, MP can be used as a biomarker of lutein and zeaxanthin in human brain tissue. This is of interest given that a significant correlation was found between MP density and global cognitive function in healthy adults. Examination of a relationship between cognition and lutein levels in brain tissue of decedents from a population-based study of adults found that among the carotenoids, only lutein was consistently associated with a wide range of cognitive measures to include executive function, language, learning and memory. Furthermore, lutein concentrations in the brain were significantly lower in individuals with mild cognitive impairment compared to those with normal cognitive function. Lastly, in controlled trials increased lutein intakes through supplements or food sources resulted in increased MP density that was associated with an improved cognitive function. Taking all of these observations into consideration, the idea that lutein can influence cognitive function warrants further study.

FUNCTIONAL FOOD FACTORS FOR PREVENTION OF DEMENTIA

Hoyoku Nishino

Cancer Control Center, Kyoto Prefectural University of Medicine, Kyoto, 602-8566, Japan

Keywords: DHA, carotenoids, polyphenols, dementia

Background: Dementia is one of the most urgent problems in Japan. Various food factors, such as DHA, carotenoids, and polyphenols, are known to have preventive potency against dementia. In this presentation, recent progress of the evaluation of these functional food factors will be introduced.

Objective and Methods: To find the good combination of functional food factors for dementia prevention, we evaluated various possible candidates for improving potency for cognitive functions.

Results: We found that some natural carotenoids and polyphenols with mild exercise are promising to improve cognitive functions in human.

Conclusion: Our study demonstrated that combinational use of some functional food factors with mild exercise may be valuable to prevent against dementia.

SULFORAPHANE AMELIORATES MEMORY DEFICITS IN A TRIPLE-TRANSGENIC MOUSE MODEL OF ALZHEIMER'S DISEASE: ITS EFFECTS ON BRAIN-DERIVED NEUROTROPHIC FACTOR EXPRESSION

Jiyoung Kim[1,2], Jisung Kim[1], Siyoung Lee[1], Bo-Ryoung Choi[3], Jung-Soo Han[3], and Ki Won Lee[1]

[1]Center for Food and Bioconvergence, Seoul National University, Seoul 08826, Republic of Korea; [2]Research Institute for Veterinary Science, College of Veterinary Medicine, Seoul National University, Seoul 08826, Republic of Korea; [3]Department of Biological Sciences, Konkuk University, Seoul 05029, Republic of Korea

Keywords: sulforaphane, memory, Alzheimer's disease, BDNF, synaptic proteins

Background: Sulforaphane, an organosulfur compound present in cruciferous vegetables, has been shown to exert neuroprotective effects in experimental *in vitro* and *in vivo* models of neurodegeneration. The brains of Alzheimer's disease (AD) patients contain low levels of brain-derived neurotrophic factor (BDNF), a neurotrophin that regulates learning and memory. BDNF has been suggested as a target protein to treat AD and ameliorate age-related brain dysfunction. Therefore, we investigated whether sulforaphane regulates BDNF expression and affects memory in a mouse model of AD.

Objective: To determine whether sulforaphane regulates BDNF expression and affects memory, we examined its effects in a mouse model of AD.

Methods: We utilized the triple transgenic mouse model of AD (3×Tg-AD), which harbors presenilin 1 (PS1, M146V), Swedish mutant amyloid precursor protein (APP, KM670/671NL), and tau (P301L) transgenes. 3×Tg-AD has been noted to have the highest face and construct validity of AD. The effects of sulforaphane on BDNF expression, levels of neuronal and synaptic molecules (microtubule-associated protein 2 [MAP-2], synaptophysin, and postsynaptic density protein-95 [PSD-95]), and BDNF-synaptic pathway components (p-tyrosine kinase receptor B [p-TrkB], p-cAMP-responsive element-binding protein [p-CREB], p-Ca^{2+}/calmodulin-dependent protein kinase II [p-CaMKII], p-Akt, and p-extracellular signal-regulated kinase [p-ERK]) were investigated in 3×Tg-AD. The effects of sulforaphane on learning and memory function were measured by novel object/location recognition and contextual fear conditioning tests.

Results: We found that oral administration of sulforaphane (10 or 50 mg/kg, 6 days a week for 8 weeks) increased BDNF levels in the cortex and hippocampus of 3×Tg-AD. Sulforaphane-treated transgenic mice also displayed increased levels of neuronal and synaptic proteins MAP-2, synaptophysin, and PSD-95. Sulforaphane elevated levels of BDNF-synaptic pathway components, p-TrkB, p-CREB, p-CaMKII, p-Akt, and p-ERK. Finally, sulforaphane ameliorated memory deficits in 3×Tg-AD.

Conclusion: These findings suggest that sulforaphane increases synaptic activity and enhances cognitive function by increasing BDNF expression in a mouse model of AD.

ACUTE RESVERATROL CONSUMPTION IMPROVES CEREBROVASCULAR RESPONSIVENESS DURING A WORKING MEMORY TASK IN ADULTS WITH TYPE 2 DIABETES

Rachel Wong, Rhenan Nealon, and Peter Howe

Clinical Nutrition Research Centre, School of Biomedical Sciences and Pharmacy, University of Newcastle, Callaghan, New South Wales 2308, Australia

Keywords: resveratrol, diabetes, transcranial Doppler ultrasound, cognition

Background: Associations between type 2 diabetes mellitus (T2DM) and accelerated cognitive decline may be attributable to the poor cerebral perfusion caused by microvascular dysfunction in T2DM. We have previously reviewed the implications of impaired working memory on everyday functioning for T2DM adults; namely the importance of working memory for self-management behaviours of their disease and the risk of falls in the elderly diabetics. We and others have shown that resveratrol consumption improves vasodilator function in the brachial artery and cerebral perfusion.

Objective: To determine the optimal dose of resveratrol to enhance cognitive performance and cerebrovascular responsiveness (CVR) during cognitive tasks in T2DM.

Methods: In a double-blind, placebo-controlled crossover intervention trial, 34 dementia-free, non-insulin dependent T2DM adults aged 40-80 years were randomised to consume a single dose of synthetic trans-resveratrol (0, 75, 150, 300mg) at weekly intervals. Transcranial Doppler ultrasound was used to assess CVR to a cognitive test battery in the middle cerebral artery at 55 and 85 min after consumption of resveratrol. Participants performed a fingertapping task during the Trial Making Test and Serial

Subtraction 3s (SS3) to assess their ability to dual-task; they also undertook a computerised multi-tasking test battery that required them to attend to four tasks simultaneously. Performance was determined as percentage accuracy. CVR to cognitive tasks was calculated as the percent increase from pre-test basal to peak mean blood flow velocity.

Results: Compared to the placebo, consumption of 75mg and 150mg resveratrol significantly increased the overall CVR to the cognitive test battery (75mg: $5.0\pm1.5\%$, $P=0.002$; 150mg: $4.7\pm1.4\%$, $P=0.002$; 300mg: $2.4\pm1.3\%$, $P=0.062$; repeated measures ANOVA). CVR during finger tapping and the SS3 was significantly enhanced following consumption of the 300mg dose ($6.4\pm2.4\%$, $P=0.012$). This enhancement was accompanied by an improvement in task performance ($4.4\pm1.7\%$ greater than placebo, $P=0.016$). However, this cognitive enhancement along with other changes in task performance or CVR to individual tasks versus placebo was no longer significant after adjusting for multiple comparisons.

Conclusion: Acute consumption of 75mg and 150mg resveratrol were equally effective in augmenting cerebral blood flow to brain regions during cognitive activation. This study also indicates that a single dose of resveratrol can acutely improve cognitive performance in adults with T2DM (a population who are known to have endothelial dysfunction and sub-clinical cognitive impairment). We must now evaluate the potential of regular resveratrol supplementation to maintain optimal cognitive functioning in other cognitive domains that have been implicated in diabetes.

Part 10
The Effects of Nutrition and Functional Foods on Ageing and Health

GENERAL LACK OF CORRELATIONS BETWEEN AGE AND SIGNS OF METABOLIC SYNDROME IN SUBJECTS WITH NON-DIABETIC FASTING GLUCOSE LEVELS

Harry G. Preuss[1], Nate Mrvichin[2], Dallas Clouatre[3], Debasis Bagchi[4], Jeffrey M Preuss[5], Nicholas V Perricone[6], and Gilbert R Kaats[2]

[1]Department of Biochemistry, Georgetown University Medical Center, Washington, D.C. 20057, USA; [2]Integrative Health Technologies, San Antonio, TX 78209, USA; [3]Glykon Technologies, Seattle, Washington 98109, USA; [4]Department of Pharmacological and Pharmaceutical Services, University of Houston, Houston, TX 77204, USA; [5]Emergency Department, Veterans Administration Medical Center, Salem, VA 24153, USA; [6]Michigan State University College of Human Medicine, East Lansing, MI 48824-136, USA

Keywords: aging, insulin resistance, metabolic syndrome

Background: Insulin resistance and chronological aging are well-accepted risk factors for the metabolic syndrome. We recently reported that fasting glucose levels in non-diabetic individuals, mirroring insulin resistance, correlate significantly in an appropriate fashion with certain elements of the metabolic syndrome suggesting a cause-effect. However, we did not examine correlations between age and many facets of the syndrome using similar methodology.

Objective: Our first goal was to determine in non-diabetic subjects (fasting glucose ≤ 125 mg/dl) with a wide age range whether significant relationships exist between chronological aging and various elements of the metabolic syndrome. Secondarily, we wished to establish if glucose-insulin metabolism is involved in influencing effects of age on the syndrome.

Methods: We gathered baseline data from 288 subjects with fasting glucose levels $\leq$ 125 mg/dl and a 17-87 year age range. Correlations between age and different metabolic parameters were assessed to determine any significant relationships and compare these with previously obtained correlations with fasting glucose levels.

Results: With the exception of a positive correlation with systolic BP, the following correlations between age and components linked to the metabolic syndrome were not significant or even significant in the opposite direction compared to correlations using fasting glucose as the independent variable: body weight, body fat, diastolic BP, WBC/neutrophil count, and circulating levels of insulin, HDL-cholesterol, triglycerides, hsCRP, ALT, and AST.

Outcome: Between ages 17-87 years, the proclivity of aging individuals possessing non-diabetic glucose levels to increase the number and breadth of correlations with adverse elements comprising the metabolic syndrome was relatively weak or did not occur. Keeping our recent findings in mind, this may be due to the fact that on an average fasting circulating glucose levels and total body fat influencing the state of insulin resistance decreased rather than increased significantly in the oldest subjects under investigation. Nevertheless, systolic BP still increased, although to a lesser extent than previously, and glomerular filtration rate decreased in the elderly despite little apparent relationship with glucose-insulin perturbations.

Conclusion: With this information in hand, it would seem wise to maintain relatively normal levels of circulating fasting glucose and insulin, i.e., avoid insulin resistance, even that appearing relatively mild, in order to avoid or lessen many future chronic health disturbances. It is important to point out, nevertheless, that the well-recognized decrease in renal glomerular filtration rate over the life cycle occurred despite the lack of more than mild age-related insulin resistance.

THE EFFICACY OF JAPANESE TRADITIONAL HERBAL MEDICINE FOR ELDERLY PATIENTS, ON NOCTURIA DUE TO NIGHT-TIME AWAKENING

Tomohiro Matsuo, Yuichiro Nakamura, Takuji Yasuda, Akihiro Asai, Kojiro Ohba, Yasuyoshi Miyata, Hideki Sakai

Department of Urology, Nagasaki University Graduate School of Biomedical Sciences, Nagasaki, Japan

Keywords: nocturia, Japanese traditional herb, overactive bladder

Background: Lower urinary symptoms can be divided into urinary storage symptoms, voiding symptoms, and post-micturition symptoms. Nocturia is a urinary storage symptom that has a considerable impact on the quality of life of both men and women affected by it. It can be caused by various factors including night-time awakening. Western sleep medicines are often prescribed for patients with nocturia due to night-time awakening. However, the use of sleep medicines, particularly in elderly patients, is a concern because of the risk of drug dependence and incidence of adverse effects such as muscle relaxation.

Kampo is a traditional herbal medicine commonly used in Japan. And we sometimes prescribe a Kampo medicine (X), which contains Angelica acutiloba, Atractylodes lancea, Bupleurum falcatum, Poria cocos, Glycyrrhiza uralensis, Cnidium officinale and Uncaria rhynchophylla, because of its efficacy in preventing difficulty in the initiation and maintenance of sleep, as well as its safety profile. However, there is no report regarding the efficacy of traditional herbal medicine on nocturia due to night-time awakening.

Objective: The aim of this study was to examine the efficacy of Japanese herbal Kampo medicine on nocturia caused by night-time awakening.

Methods: Consent was obtained from patients admitted to our facility for nocturia due to night-time awakening. Patients with a neurogenic bladder, urinary tract infection, or urological malignant tumor were excluded. The participants were treated with 2.5 g of the X three times a day for 12 weeks. Drugs used for the improvement of urinary function and sleep that were administered before participation in this study were not changed during the study. Overactive bladder symptom score (OABSS) and hours of undisturbed sleep (HUS) prior to the first awakening were determined before treatment and 12 weeks after treatment to evaluate the efficacy using the Pittsburgh sleep quality index (PSQI). A P value of less than 0.05 was considered to indicate statistical significance.

Results: Twenty-four patients (12 male and 12 female) with a mean age of 74.4 ± 9.8 years participated in this study after giving consent. While 3 patients complained of difficulty in swallowing the drug because of its bitterness, all patients completed this study without any particular adverse event. The total OABSS decreased from 4.6 ± 1.7 (before treatment) to 2.8 ± 1.9 (after treatment) ($P < 0.001$), while night-time frequency decreased from 2.6 ± 0.6 to 1.8 ± 0.9 ($P < 0.001$). The actual number of night-time voiding reduced from 3.7 ± 2.2 times to 2.2 ± 1.8 times ($P < 0.001$).
Interestingly, the score for daytime frequency also decreased from 0.5 ± 0.7 to 0.2 ± 0.4 ($P = 0.049$). Furthermore, the actual number of daytime urinary frequency reduced from 7.4 ± 2.1 times to 6.1 ± 1.7 times ($P = 0.002$). In addition, urgency also significantly improved ($P = 0.003$). HUS prolonged from 2.4 ± 0.6 hours to 3.3 ± 1.2 hours ($P = 0.002$) and PSQI decreased from 7.6 ± 3.1 to 5.7 ± 1 ($P < 0.001$).

Conclusion: The efficacy of the X in patients with nocturia due to night-time awakening was confirmed. Although the study subjects were relatively old, treatment with the X successfully improved the quality of sleep without causing major side effects. Moreover, administration of the X improved daytime urinary frequency and urgency. Thus, further clinical investigation including application to OAB is desired in the future.

Part 11
Roles of Food Derived Nitrite / Nitrate from Cured Meat to Vegetables, to Hypertension and/or Antioxidant Effect

WHAT IS THE ROLE OF INORGANIC NITRATE AND NITRITE IN CARDIOVASCULAR DISEASE: A SYSTEMATIC REVIEW OF HUMAN EVIDENCE

Jacklyn Jackson[1], Lesley MacDonald-Wicks[2], Amanda Patterson[2], Mark McEvoy[3]

[1]School of Health Sciences, Faculty of Health and Medicine, University of Newcastle, University Drive, Callaghan, NSW, Australia; [2]Priority Research Centre in Physical Activity and Nutrition, University of Newcastle, NSW, Australia; [3]Centre for Clinical Epidemiology and Biostatistics, Hunter Medical Research Institute, University of Newcastle, Callaghan, NSW, 2308, Australia.

Keywords: inorganic nitrate, inorganic nitrite, cardiovascular disease, systematic review, humans

Background: Cardiovascular disease (CVD) is the leading cause of mortality worldwide and inadequate Nitric Oxide (NO) bioavailability is thought to play a major role in CVD pathogenesis. Nitric oxide is a key signaling molecule in the cardiovascular system acting primarily as a potent vasodilator. Inorganic nitrate and nitrite can be metabolized in the body to produce NO via the Nitrate-Nitrite-NO pathway. Vegetables (especially beetroot and green leafy vegetables) provide the richest source of dietary inorganic nitrate; however, their role in preventing or treating CVD via their NO donor activity remains uncertain.

Objective: This systematic review aimed to investigate the effect of inorganic nitrate and nitrite on CVD risk factors and outcomes in humans.

Methods: Five electronic databases (Medline, Embase, CINAHL, Cochrane and Scopus) were systematically searched for published studies that included adults ($\geq$18 years) and investigated the effect of inorganic nitrate intake in relation to various CVD outcomes (e.g. All-cause mortality, Myocardial Infarction, atherosclerosis) and risk factors (e.g. changes in blood lipids, blood pressure and arterial stiffness).

Results: Fifty-four articles were included for review containing a total of 60 relevant interventions. Fifty-seven of the interventions were randomized controlled trials; two were controlled before and after studies and one a case series study. A total of 1094 participants were included, and intervention lengths ranged from one hour to 70 days in duration. None of the included studies investigated CVD outcomes, instead only CVD risk factors such as blood pressure, endothelial function, arterial stiffness, blood lipids and platelet aggregation were studied. Evidence from this review indicates some utility of inorganic nitrate and nitrite intakes for improved blood pressures, endothelial function and arterial stiffness in humans.

Conclusion: It remains unclear if there is an optimum dose or form of inorganic nitrate/nitrite intake required to reduce risk of CVD events within the general adult population. In addition, this review indicates a clear need for more long-term evidence to determine if inorganic nitrate and nitrite intakes reduce risk of cardiovascular disease outcomes, as it could provide evidence for a relatively simple and low cost public health intervention option for reducing CVD burden in the population.

DIETARY NITRITE AND NITRATE: FROM MENACE TO MARVEL

Nathan S. Bryan

Baylor College of Medicine, Houston, TX USA

Dietary sources of nitrite and nitrate were once considered toxic food additives that contributed to endogenous nitrosamine formation and thus there were enormous efforts to limit exposure. However, very consistent and compelling biomedical research over the past 15 years has revealed that these two anions may actually have health promoting effects. There are now indisputable health benefits of nitrite and nitrate derived from food sources or when administered in a clinical setting for specific diseases. Most of the published reports identify the production of nitric oxide (NO) as the mechanism of action for nitrite and nitrate. Basic science as well as clinical studies demonstrates nitrite and/or nitrate can restore NO homeostasis as an endothelium independent source of NO that may be a redundant system for endogenous NO production. Nitrate must first be reduced to nitrite by oral commensal bacteria and then nitrite further reduced to NO along the physiological oxygen gradient.

The objective of this presentation review is to define their role as indispensable nutrients needed for maintaining NO homeostasis and describe the daily intake required in order to achieve a threshold of activation as well as define the upper tolerable limits based on published literature in PubMed databases. Optimal ranges of intake will be discussed in order to maximize the benefits while mitigating any potential risks of overexposure to these naturally occurring anions. This information will allow for future research using safe and effective doses of nitrite and nitrate in long term clinical trials in order to effectively test their roles in disease prevention or treatment. Defining the context for the benefits for nitrite and nitrate while mitigating risk of nitrosamine formation may define new guidelines for optimal health.

LEARNING OBJECTIVES:
1. Understand the role of nitric oxide in health and disease
2. Define the mechanism of dietary nitrate and nitrite reduction to NO in the human body
3. Understand the nutrient value of nitrite and nitrate and how diets rich in these anions can prevent and treat many contemporary diseases

ARABINOXYLAN EXTRACTS FOR IMMUNITY: MODULATION PATHWAY

Weili Li[1], Zhengxiao Zhang[2], Christopher Smith[1], Jason Ashworth[3]

[1]Institute of Food Science and Innovation, University of Chester, Chester, CH1 4BJ, UK; [2]Department of Food and Tourism Management, Manchester Metropolitan University, Manchester, M15 6BG, UK; [3]School of Healthcare Science, Manchester Metropolitan University, Manchester, M1 5GD, UK

Keywords: Arabinoxylans, Molecular structures, Immuno-modulatory activity, Nitric oxide, Inducible nitric oxide synthase, U937 cells

Background: Arabinoxylans (AXs) are an important group of hemicelluloses found in the outer-layer and endosperm cell walls of cereals and have been reported to possess various biological activities, such as immunity enhancement, antioxidant activity, post-prandial glycaemic response reduction, and lowering serum cholesterol. Therefore, the previous results demonstrated that AXs can be considered a potential bioactive food supplement. The recent study of our research group on the relationship between immunomodulating ability and the various structures of AXs encourage continued investigation into the structure-activity relationship of AXs and possible immune modulation mechanism.

Objective: To further examine the immunomodulatory activity and study possible modulation pathways in relation to AX molecular structures. AXs, with various molecular structures, were investigated to determine the relationship(s) between their structure and immunomodulatory activity using a human macrophage cell line, U937, to measure cell viability, growth and nitric oxide (NO) production. Furthermore, the interactions between AXs and inducible nitric oxide synthase (iNOS) expression were also tested to analyse the possible mechanisms involved.

Methods: The Human U937 macrophage cells were incubated with medium containing 10-1000 µg/mL of water extracted AXs (WEAX) and enzyme degraded AXs (E-WEAX) respectively, with lipopolysaccharide (LPS) as a positive control. We measured cell viability, growth and NO release from U937 cells using Griess' reagent. Under the same conditions, the expressions of iNOS were also analysed using Dot blot assay.

Results: The present study indicated AX samples have no inhibitory effects on the viability and cell growth of the human U937 macrophage, even at 1000µg/ml. The two AXs sample treatments over the concentration range from 1 to 500µg/ml significantly elevated NO production by U937 cells after a 24h incubation period compared with the untreated control ($p < 0.05$). Furthermore, the amount of NO production significantly increased at 10µg/ml of E-WEAX treatment compared to the lower concentrations ($p < 0.05$). However, there was a significant decrease in NO secretion following E-WEAX treatment at 500µg/ml ($p < 0.05$) compared to that at 50µg/ml. Unlike E-WEAX treatment, there was a general NO secretion increase by WEAX treatment till the concentration was up to 500µg/ml compared lower concentrations 1-10µg/ml treatments ($p < 0.1$), suggesting the peak amount of NO released by the WEAX treatment may have not reached yet. Hence, these results indicate that there is a possibly optimal dose of E-WEAX for NO production in the range 10-50µg/ml whilst WEAX has a significant different optimum dose above 500µg/ml. In addition, in the concentration range from 10 to 50µg/ml, NO response of WEAX is much more modest than that produced by similar concentrations of E-WEAX ($p < 0.05$). Thus, these comparisons show there are obvious differences between E-

WEAX and WEAX treatments in relation to NO stimulation and WEAX had generally weaker NO stimulation activity than E-WEAX in the present assay. LPS was used as a positive control and significantly stimulated NO secretion at concentrations of 1 to 50μg/ml compared to the untreated control, which is similar to E-WEAX. However, at 500μg/ml of LPS, the amount of NO produced by the U937 cells significantly decreased ($p<0.05$) compared to lower concentrations of LPS, reflecting the substantial inhibitory effect on cell growth and viability at this concentration. Compared with AXs, the NO produced following LPS treatment is consistently higher than that produced by WEAX at concentrations of 1 to 50μg/ml ($p<0.05$). Interestingly, there was no significant difference between the amount of NO produced with E-WEAX and LPS treatments at concentrations at and above 10 μg/ml ($p>0.05$), suggesting E-WEAX was equally effective at NO stimulation as LPS at these concentrations. In addition, WEAX and E-WEAX significantly elevated the level of iNOS expression by U937 cells after a 24h incubation period compared with the control ($p<0.05$). However, the amount of iNOS following treatment with E-WEAX was significantly higher than with WEAX ($p<0.05$). LPS was used as a positive control and it presented a significant increase in iNOS expression compared to control ($p<0.05$). There was no significant difference between LPS and the two AX samples in terms of iNOS concentration in U937 cell lysates ($p>0.05$) at the same treatment concentration. It is obvious that the stimulatory effect of AXs on iNOS induction is highly correlated with their stimulatory activity on NO production. Therefore, the increased NO production by AXs treatment was possibly due to induced levels of iNOS by U937 cells. The LPS (positive control) also showed a high stimulatory activity on iNOS levels in U937 cell lysates in the testing

Conclusion: The analysis of the relationship between the molecular structures and the immunomodulatory activity of AX samples in in vitro testing suggests differences in the stimulatory effect on NO secretion are closely associated with the enzyme modified AXs which have a much higher proportion of lower Mw AXs and higher A/X ratio than the non-enzyme treated AXs. Furthermore, the effects of AXs on iNOS levels of human macrophage cells positively related to the increase in NO secretion, which suggest a pathway by which AXs modulate NO production in human macrophage cells.

Part 12
Functional Foods with Bioactive Compound(s): Prevention and Management of Noncommunicable Diseases

EFFECTS OF GRAPE WINE AND APPLE CIDER VINEGAR ON OXIDATIVE AND ANTIOXIDATIVE STATUS IN HIGH CHOLESTEROL-FED RATS

Atıf Can Seydim[1], Zeynep Banu Güzel-Seydim[1], Duygu Kumbul Doğuç[2], M. Çağrı Savaş[3], Havva Nilgün Budak[4]

[1]Suleyman Demirel University, Department of Food Engineering, Isparta, Turkey; [2]Suleyman Demirel University, Department of Medical Biochemistry, Faculty of Medicine, Isparta, Turkey; [3]SuleymanDemirel University, Department of Pediatric Surgery, Faculty of Medicine, Isparta, Turkey; [4]Suleyman Demirel University, Department of Food Processing, Egirdir Vocational School, Isparta, Turkey

Keywords: Oxidative stress, grape vinegar, apple cider vinegar, glutathione peroxidase (GSH-Px), superoxide dismutase (SOD), malondialdehyde (MDA), catalase (CAT), high-cholesterol-fed rat

Background: Oxidative stress is the result of an imbalance between the rates of free radical production and elimination via endogenous antioxidant mechanisms such as antioxidant enzymes; glutathione peroxidase (GSH-Px), superoxide dismutase (SOD), catalase (CAT). Antioxidants widely available in fruits, vegetables, and seeds have been shown to possess a broad spectrum of biological, pharmacological and therapeutic properties against oxidative stress. Consumption of fruits and vegetables are essential as much as their products such as fruit juices, wines and vinegars, which contain significant amount of polyphenolic compounds. Vinegar is produced mainly from different varieties of wine by two fermentation step, ethanol and acetic acid fermentations. Followed by wine production, there are mainly two vinegar production methods. One is surface also known as traditional method. The second method is submerging technique involving submerged culture where the oxygenation has been greatly improved (industrial method).

Objective: The aim of the study is to determine the effects of grape and apple cider vinegar consumption against oxidative stress in high cholesterol-fed rats.

Methods: Fifty-four male adult Wistar albino rats were included in the study. Rats were divided into six groups of nine. 1 mL of 2.5% cholesterol (at 5pm) and 1 mL of different vinegar samples (at 9am) were administered daily for 7 weeks by oral gavage; Control-diet group (CNT) received 1mL of normal saline solution concurrently with the experiment groups. Rats were sacrificed at the end of the experiment and blood samples were collected. The erythrocyte samples were washed three times in normal saline (0.9%, v/w) and then hemolyzed with 2mL of cold bidistillated water. CAT activity was measured following the method of Aebi. MDA was determined by the double heating method of Draper and Hadley. GSH-Px activity was measured according to the method of Paglia and Valentine. SOD activity was analyzed according to the method of Woolliams et al. (1983). Both were analyzed in Beckmann Coulter AU 5800 auto analyzer by using RANDOX kits (Randox Laboratories Ltd. Ardmore, Crumlin, UK).

Vinegars were obtained after the grape and apple vinegar fermentations using surface culture method and industrial submerge methods. Grape and apple juices were immediately inoculated with *Saccharomyces cerevisiae* (0.02%) for ethanol fermentation for 30 days at 25°C. After the completion of the ethanol fermentation, acetic acid fermentation of the wines was initiated with the addition of two-year aged vinegar (1:3 ratio) using surface technique at 25°C and continued for 60 days at 25°C. Vinegars produced by the industrial submerge method for 24 hours at 25°C were transported to the Department of Food Engineering laboratories from the Carl Kuhne Vinegar Plant located in

Afyonkarahisar, Turkey. Total antioxidant activity of vinegar samples were measured by Oxygen Radical Absorbance Capacity (ORAC) and 2,2'-azinobis (3-ethlybenzthiazoline)-6-sulfonic acid (ABTS) methods.

Results: Levels of CAT, GSH-Px, SOD of CHOLCNT group were significantly decreased while MDA levels were significantly increased when compared to CNT group. Levels of MDA which is the end-product of lipid peroxidation was significantly decreased in the apple cider vinegar administered groups (AVS and AVM) when compared to the CHOLCNT (P<0.05). MDA levels of grape wine vinegar administered groups were decreased (GVS, GVM); however, the difference was not significant. GSH-Px levels were significantly increased in both GVS and AVS groups, which were fed with the vinegars produced by traditional surface methods. (P=0.03, P=0.001 respectively) compared to the CHOLCNT. GSH-Px levels of rats fed with vinegars produced with industrial submerge methods (GVM, AVM), showed no significant difference when compared to CHOLCNT group. SOD levels of GVS, GVM, AVS, AVM were significantly increased as compared to CHOLCNT group (p<0.05). TEAC and ORAC values of vinegar samples (GVS and AVS) produced with surface methods were higher than other samples. ORAC and TEAC value of AVS sample was 5.89 μmol trolox/ml and 5.5 mM, respectively.

Conclusion: Present research showed that high cholesterol diet increased lipid peroxidation and consumed the antioxidant enzymes. Although the degree of the effect on antioxidant enzyme activity differs, the use of vinegar especially the ones produced by surface culture methods seem to have favorable effect *in vivo*. These findings are in concordance with the ORAC and TEAC values of vinegars.

DROUGHT STRESS AFFECTS ORGANIC AND INORGANIC BIOACTIVE COMPOUNDS IN POTATOES RELEVANT TO NON-COMMUNICABLE DISEASES (NCD)

Christina B. Wegener, Hans-Ulrich Jürgens, Gisela Jansen

Julius Kuehn Institute (JKI); Institute for Resistance Research and Stress Tolerance, Rudolf-Schick-Platz 3, 18190 Sanitz, Germany

Keywords: potato, drought stress, bioactive compounds, chronic diseases

Background: Drought is one of the main abiotic stress factors that limits productivity of crop plants and will become increasingly more important worldwide, especially in the course of climate change. The potato (*Solanum tuberosum* L.), a staple food, is highly sensitive to drought. Besides yield losses, plant stress responses may affect metabolites associated with the health value of tubers.

Objective: To evaluate the effects of drought stress on bioactive compounds relevant to human health.

Methods: One yellow-fleshed cultivar (Agave) and two purple breeding clones (St 3792, St 89403) were analyzed in the experiments carried out with four replications in a randomized design, over two years. The plants were grown in pots in a glasshouse with optimal water supply and under drought stress conditions. After tuber initiation the water supply was fully stopped for six days, and after this drought period, watering was reduced continuously from 50 ml daily per plant to 30 ml and eventually to 20 ml (2. year). In the first year, the stress was less strong with 25.4% yield loss on average than in the second year (-35.7%). After harvest, the tubers of these two variants were analyzed for health-relevant compounds like sugars, starch, minerals, crude protein, free amino acids (AAS) and fatty acids (FA) using standard analytical and statistical methods.

Results: Apart from genotypic differences in most parameters, the results revealed that drought stress lead to a decline in glucose and fructose *(P < 0.05*, all), in both years. The sucrose content increased (*P < 0.01*), especially in the second year with a stronger stress, and starch was reduced in its tendency. On the other hand, amounts of protein, GABA and AAS, above all asparagine (+49.3%) and proline (+43.8%), a stress related marker, were enhanced (*P < 0.01, all*). Moreover, drought boosted the minerals Mg, K and P (*P < 0.01, all*), whereas Ca was diminished (*P < 0.05*). The portion of α-linolenic acid (ALA), an essential FA, on total lipids was higher in drought stressed tubers (*P < 0.01*) than in well-watered control tubers, while oleic acid as its precursor decreased (*P < 0.05*). This was found for all genotypes, but only in the first year. In the second year, characterized by a severe stress (up to -47.1% yield loss) the ALA was in general higher and thus not further induced. All other FAs, including linoleic, palmitic and stearic acid were less strongly affected by drought. It is also important, that *myo*-inositol (MIS) and lipid acyl hydrolases (LAH) associated with modulation in cell membrane lipids (*P < 0.01, both*) increased by drought, in each year. MIS and LAH data detected for the stressed tubers in the second test year correlated significantly (r = 0.90, *P < 0.01*), possibly indicating a concerted action within plant stress responses. MIS can be part of membrane phospholipids and also cytosolic inositols may protect cellular structures against environmental stresses.

Conclusions: Drought stress has a clear effect on bioactive compounds of tubers. Decline in glucose and fructose, and increase in crude protein, GABA, AAS, ALA, MIS and minerals like Mg, K and P, on the other side, may be profitable for health benefits of potatoes. Relations of these biochemical changes to NCDs are worthy to be discussed, together with antioxidants studied in a previous project.

DISTRIBUTION OF POLYPHENOLS IN SOME SPECIES OF AFRICAN EGGPLANT FRUITS (*Solanum spp*) INHIBITS α-AMYLASE, α-GLUCOSIDASE AND ANGIOTENSIN-1-CONVERTING ENZYME ACTIVITIES IN-VITRO

Esther E. Nwanna, Emmanuel O. Ibukun' and Ganiyu Oboh

Functional food, Nutraceuticals and phytomedicine, Department of Biochemistry, Federal University of Technology, P.M.B 704 Akure, Nigeria

Keywords: Solanum spp, polyphenols, diabetes, enzymes

Background: *Solanum* is a common and popular vegetable crop grown in the subtropics and tropics (Sarker *et al.*, 2006). Eggplant is a perennial but grown commercially as an annual crop. The ripe fruit of eggplant is primarily used as a cooking vegetable for the various dishes all over the world. Eggplants come from various kinds of varieties, which are highly variable in fruit colour, as well as fruit shape and size.

Objectives: This study focuses on the interaction of phenolic extracts from some Nigerian eggplants *Solanum melogen depressum*, *Solanum gilo* and *Solanum melogena* with enzymes linked to type-2 diabetes (a-glucosidase and a-amylase) and hypertension [Angiotensin I converting enzyme (ACE)].

Methods: Different solvent mixtures were used to extract the phenolics from the pulp residues. Free phenolics were extracted with 80% acetone, while bound phenolics were extracted from the alkaline and acid hydrolyzed residue with ethyl acetate. The total phenolic and flavonoid content, antioxidant activities, and interaction of the extracts with a-glucosidase, a-amylase and ACE were subsequently determined.

Results: The free phenolics with the range [1.54mgGAE/g – 1.37mgGAE/g] and flavonoid [0.33mgQE/g – 0.59mgQE/g] content was significantly (P<0.05) higher than bound phenolic [0.49mgGAE/g – 0.68mgGAE/g] and flavonoid [0.l0mgQE/g – 0.26mgQE/g] content of the three eggplant species. The free and bound phenolics extracts inhibited α-glucosidase, α-amylase and ACE activities in a concentration dependent manner. Moreover, free phenolic extracts from *Solanum melogen depressum* had the highest inhibitory effect on α-amylase (EC_{50}= 79.48μg/ml) and its bound phenolic extra had the highest inhibitory effect on ACE (EC_{50}= 98.68μg/ml) activities, while bound phenolic extract from *Solanum melogen depressum* had the highest inhibitory effect on α-glucosidase (EC_{50}= 170.24μg/m1) activities. The free and bound phenolics extract exhibited antioxidant activities as typified by their ferric reducing antioxidant ability (FRAP).

Conclusion: Our studies revealed that eggplant consists of different phenolic compound and antioxidant properties. *Solanum melogen depressum* extracts had better inhibition of enzymes linked with type-2 diabetes and hypertension, which could be a result of its higher total flavonoids content and higher bound phenolics compare to the others varieties.

APPLE PEEL FLAVONOIDS AF4 INHIBIT TRIPLE NEGATIVE BREAST CANCER CELL PROLIFERATION AND MIGRATION

Wasundara Fernando[1], H.P. Vasantha Rupasinghe[1,4], and David W. Hoskin[1, 2, 3]

Departments of Pathology[1], Microbiology and Immunology[2] and Surgery[3], Faculty of Medicine, Dalhousie University, Halifax, NS, Canada; Department of Environmental Sciences[4], Faculty of Agriculture, Dalhousie University, Truro, NS, Canada

Keywords: dietary flavonoids, apple, breast cancer, cytotoxicity, metastasis

Background: Breast cancer is the most common cancer among females worldwide and accounts for 12% of all cancers diagnosed. Triple-negative breast cancer contributes for 15-20% of all invasive types of breast cancer; however, due to the lack of known specific therapeutic targets, triple-negative breast cancer has been characterized as an aggressive type of breast cancer with poor prognosis. Flavonoids are a subgroup of phytochemicals which are well-known to possess extensive health benefits, including antioxidant, anti-inflammatory and anticancer activities. Flavonoids are ubiquitously found in plant-based food. The investigation of food-derived biomolecules to treat cancer has received attention due to their potential to act as broad-spectrum cancer-targeting agents.

Objectives: To investigate the cytotoxic and antimetastatic properties of a flavonoid-rich ethanolic extract of apple peels using triple-negative and estrogen receptor-positive mammary carcinoma cells.

Methods: Cytotoxicity of the apple-derived flavonoid fraction (AF4) toward triple-negative (MDA-MB-231, MDA-MB-468 and

4T1) and estrogen receptor-positive (MCF-7 and T-47D) mammary carcinoma cells was tested and compared to human non-malignant mammary epithelial cells (HMECs and MCF-10A) using MTS assay. Flow cytometric analysis of Annexin-V-FLUOS/propidium iodide (PI)-stained MCF-10A and human dermal fibroblasts compared to MDA-MB-231 cells was performed to confirm the selective cytotoxicity of AF4 for mammary carcinoma cells. The Amplex Red assay and flow cytometric analysis of MDA-MB-231 cells treated with AF4 either in the presence or absence of N-acetylcysteine was performed to test the involvement of reactive oxygen species (ROS) in AF4-induced cell death. The ability of AF4 to induce necrotic cell death was examined by treating MDA-MB-231 cells with AF4 either in the presence or absence of necrostatin-1, a potent inhibitor of necroptosis. *In vivo* tumor suppressor properties of the intratumoral administration of AF4 was tested using MDA-MB-231 xenograft bearing non-obese diabetic severe combined immune-deficient (NOD-SCID) female mice. Wound-healing and trans-well cell migration assays were performed using MDA-MB-231 and 4T1 cells to evaluate the *in vitro* antimetastatic properties of AF4. The effect of AF4 on the expression of proteins involved in the epithelial-to-mesenchymal transition (EMT) was measured using western blot analysis of MDA-MB-231 cell lysates.

Results: The metabolic activity of triple-negative and estrogen receptor positive mammary carcinoma cell lines was decreased in a dose- and time-dependent manner following AF4 treatment. AF4 selectively killed breast cancer cells since the least cytotoxic effects were seen on non-malignant mammary epithelial cells and fibroblasts. Neither necrostatin-1 nor N-acetylcysteine was able to protect the breast cancer cells from AF4-induced cytotoxicity. AF4 also suppressed MDA-MB-231 xenograft growth in NOD-SCID mice. The migration of 4T1 and MDA-MB-231 mammary carcinoma cells was significantly suppressed by sub-cytotoxic doses of AF4 in a dose-dependent manner. The expression of EMT markers, β-catenin, slug and matrix metalloproteinase (MMP)-2 was down-regulated by AF4.

Conclusion: AF4-induced cytotoxicity is dose- and time-dependent and selective for mammary carcinoma cells. ROS production or necroptosis is not involved in AF4-induced cell death. Importantly, AF4 suppresses *in vivo* tumor progression. In addition, sub-cytotoxic doses of AF4 block the migration of mammary carcinoma cells and down-regulate the expression of EMT-associated regulatory proteins, β-catenin, slug and MMP-2. These observations suggest that AF4 can be developed as a selective cytotoxic natural health product to treat triple negative breast cancer progression and metastasis.

BOVINE LACTOFERRIN PROMOTE THE PROLIFERATION OF OSTEOBLAST TO PREVENT OSTEOPOROSIS

Jiliang Zhang[1], Lanwei Zhang[1] *, Xue Han[1], and Huaxi Yi[1]

[1]School of Chemistry and Chemical Engineering, Harbin Institute of Technology, Harbin, 150080, China

Keywords: bovine lactoferrin, osteoblast, osteoporosis, proliferation

Background: Osteoporosis is a disease that causes significant bone loss, micro-architectural deterioration and degradation of macroscopic bone properties. Bone lining cells, osteoblasts and osteocytes, have been proposed to act as mechanosensors within bone tissue. Lactoferrin (LF) is a natural component of milk, and as a pleiotropic factor and involves many biological processes, such as: regulation of levels of free iron in the body fluids, immunoregulation, anti-tumor, anti-microbial and anti-virus. Bovine LF (bLF) has been reported as a growth factor that can stimulate the proliferation and protect apoptosis of osteoblast cells to prevent the osteoporosis, but natural human LF (hLF) belonging to same family is lacking in understanding.

Objective: To evaluate the cell proliferation effect on osteoblast between bLF and natural hLF, and provide theoretical basis for follow-up bLF exploiting in formula food and healthy food to prevent osteoporosis.

Methods: The osteoblast cell line, the MC3T3-E1subclone 14, was incubated with medium of α-MEM containing 10% FBS, 1% penicillin-streptomycin. For subculture, cells at 90% confluence were passaged after detachment in 0.25% trypsin. We measured the proliferation effects of bLF and hLF by MTT, the prevent apoptosis effects of bLF and hLF by CCK-8 kit, secretion of alkaline phosphatase by ALP kit, and Flow cytometry to measure the cell cycle. Furthermore, we studied the expressions of mRNA associated with proliferating cell nuclear antigen (PCNA) by RT-PCR, and also the PCNA expression by western blotting. hLF and bLF with concentrations of 1, 10 and 100 mg/L treated for 24, 48 and 72 h.

Results: 100 mg/L both of bLF and hLF promoted the proliferation of osteoblasts, and sustained osteoblasts at the highest survival rate at 48 h compared with control and improved the G2/M and S phage for 48 and 72 h, but bLF performed significant difference ($P < 0.05$) compared with hLF. 100 mg/L bLF treated for 48 h significantly ($P < 0.05$) increased the secretion of ALP compared with the control. Grey analysis showed that the expression of mRNA and PCNA treated by bLF and hLF were significantly ($P < 0.05$) higher than control, and the expression by bLF significantly higher than hLF ($P < 0.05$). These results indicated that bLF had better effects on cell proliferation of MC3T3-E1 compared with hLF.

Conclusion: Our study demonstrated that bovine lactoferrin and human lactoferrin both can promote the proliferative, increase the secretion of alkaline phosphatase, shortage the cell cycle of MC3T3-E1, increase the mRNA and protein expression of PCNA. Lactoferrin may play an important role in prevention of osteoporosis. Bovine lactoferrin had better proliferation effects than human lactoferrin at the same concentration and treating time.

ANGIOTENSIN I CONVERTING ENZYME INHIBITORY PROPERTIES OF ENZYMATIC YAK MILK CASEIN HYDROLYSATES

Kai Lin[1], Lanwei Zhang[1], Xue Han[1], Huaxi Yi[1], Dayou Cheng[1]

[1]School of Chemistry and Chemical Engineering, Harbin Institute of Technology, Harbin, 150000, China

Keywords: ACE inhibitory activity, yak milk casein hydrolysates, enzymatic hydrolysis

Background: Hypertension is one of the major public health problems worldwide and poses a main risk factor for cardiovascular disease complications such as coronary heart disease, stroke, congestive heart failure, heart rhythm irregularities and kidney failure, etc. Angiotensin I converting enzyme (dipeptidyl carboxypeptidase, EC 3.4.15.1, ACE) plays a critical role in regulating blood pressure by virtue of the renin–angiotensin system (RAS) and kallikrein kinnin system (KKS). Therefore, inhibition of ACE activity can contribute to lowering blood pressure. Recently, many ACE inhibitory peptides derived from food proteins were reported, as natural alternative bioactive peptides are milder and safer than synthetic ACE inhibitors. Yak milk, the major ingredients of the daily diets of Tibetan herders, are widely used in the production of butter, and the by-product (Qula, a kind of crude cheese, whose main component is casein) is not fully used. Furthermore, the amino acid composition of yak milk casein are very similar to that of cow milk, thus it is a suitable resource for the generation of ACE inhibitory peptides.

Objective: In the present study, various types of enzyme were used to hydrolyze yak milk casein for preparing peptide mixtures and to investigate the effect of protease type on the ACE-inhibitory activities of hydrolysates.

Methods: Yak milk casein was hydrolyzed by six different enzymes (alcalase, thermolysin, proteinase K, trypsin, papain and α-chymotrypsin). The degree of hydrolysis of the hydrolysates, which indicates the extent of the protein degradation, was measured during the whole reaction process. The tricine-SDS-PAGE was also used to explore the molecular weight distribution of hydrolysates. To know the most effective condition to obtain ACE inhibitory peptides, ACE inhibitory activities of hydrolysates versus the hydrolysis times were measured. Then, the hydrolysates possessed high ACE inhibitory activity was passed through a 3kDa regenerated cellulose ultra-filtration membranes and their IC_{50} was calculated. In addition, the mass fingerprints of 3kDa permeate from hydrolysates were analyzed by matrix-assisted laser desorption/ionization time of flight mass (MAIDI-TOF-MS) spectrometry. Finally, the inhibitory kinetics of yak milk casein hydrolysates (<3 kDa fraction) with most potent activity were investigated.

Results: The degree of hydrolysis of six proteases exhibited an initial fast reaction rate after the addition of each enzyme, and then followed by a slowdown which reached a plateau where no apparent hydrolysis took place at 50 min for α-chymotrypsin (11.27 %[a]), 90 min for thermolysin(18.97 %[b]), 120 min for alcalase (21.90 %[c]), 150 min for papain (29.71 %[d]) and 210 min for proteinase K, trypsin(23.86 %[c], 18.50 %[b]) ($P<0.05$). According to the electrophoretic profiles, complete degradation of yak milk casein was only achieved after 10 min of treatment with all the using enzymes, and then degraded gradually. After digestion, the hydrolysates of yak milk casein showed potent ACE inhibitory activities. We found that the hydrolysates showed ACE inhibitory activities from the first 30 min of digestion. The ACE-inhibitory activities of thermolysin (83.41 %), alcalase (79.15 %) and papain (72.11 %) treated hydrolysates were relatively higher than others and reached a plateau from 60 to 240min of hydrolysis (P<0.05). The ACE-inhibitory activities of proteinase K (64.58 %) treated hydrolysates gradually increased during the whole hydrolysis process. In the case of trypsin (63.19 %) treated hydrolysates, the ACE inhibitory activities increased in the early stages of hydrolysis and then decreased slightly. α-Chymotrypsin (44.15%) treated hydrolysates showed the lowest ACE inhibitory activity. Comparing the two molecular weight fractions of enzymatic hydrolysates reveals that the highest ACE inhibitory activity was exhibited by thermolysin treated hydrolysates lower than 3 kDa(IC$_{50}$ 0.1313 mg/mL), and a total of 26 peptides have been identified with molecular weights ranging from 200 to 3000 kDa by MAIDI-TOF-MS. The inhibitory kinetic property of thermolysin treated hydrolysates was evaluated by Lineweaver–Burk curve and found to be noncompetitive. It also has the lowest inhibition constant (K$_i$) 0.2091 mg/mL, which indicates greater affinity between peptide and ACE protein.

Conclusion: Our study demonstrated that yak milk casein would be an attractive raw material for the production of ACE inhibitory peptides. Yak milk casein hydrolysates treated by alcalase, thermolysin, proteinase K, trypsin and papain except α-chymotrypsin showed relatively high ACE inhibitory activity in vitro. In addition, the hydrolysates filtered through 3kDa ultra-filtration membrane showed the low molecular weight fraction had higher ACE inhibitory activity than that of the high molecular weight. Finally, we found that incubation with thermolysin produced the most active peptides and brought about the lowest IC_{50} value. Furthermore, the identified peptides obtained by thermolysin showed a sequence that could explain the high ACE inhibitory activity. Therefore, the present study suggests that yak milk casein can be utilized for developing high value-added functional foods.

THE ELUCIDATION OF THE MECHANISM OF LENTINAN-INDUCED INFLAMMATORY SUPPRESSION BY VISUALIZING TNFR1 ON THE MEMBRANE

Kana Sakaguchi[1], Takashi Hashimoto[1], Toshiki Itoh[2], Yasuhito Shirai[1], and Masashi Mizuno[1]

[1]Department of Agrobioscience, Graduate School of Agricultural Science, Kobe University, Kobe, 657-8501, Japan; [2]Biosignal Research Center, Organization of Advanced Science and Technology, Kobe University, Kobe, 657-8501, Japan

Keywords: lentinan, intestinal inflammation, IEC, TNFR1

Background: Lentinan, β-1,3-1,6- glucan extracted from *Lentinula edodes*, has been shown to suppress the intestinal inflammation *in vivo* and *in vitro* gut inflammatory models. The gut inflammatory is induced by IL-8 production from intestinal epithelium cells (IECs) via the TNF-α receptor 1 (TNFR1) - mediated NF-κB activation, resulting in the migration of neutrophils into the inflamed site. The previous study demonstrated that lentinan was recognized by the dectin-1 on the surface of epithelial cells and decreased TNFR1 expressed on basal membrane of IECs. However, it is unclear how lentinan regulates the amount of TNFR1 on the cell membrane.

Objective: To elucidate the mechanism to regulate of TNFR1 expression on cell membrane by lentinan, the plasmid encoding TNFR1 and green fluorescent protein (GFP) fusion protein was transfected into the intestinal cell line Caco-2 cells, and the effect of lentinan on TNFR1 on the membrane was monitored.

Methods: We produced plasmids encoding several types of TNFR1 and GFP. The plasmid was transfected into Caco-2 cells, seeded onto glass bottom dishes by lipofection. The cells were incubated with the lentinan solution (500 μg/ml) for 6 hours and the TNFR1 on the membrane (membrane-TNFR1) was labelled with anti-TNFR1 antibody, followed by immunofluorescence staining with Alexa594-conjugated secondary antibody. Both GFP and Alexa594 were observed under confocal laser scanning microscope (CLFM). The movement of membrane-TNFR1 at one molecular level was elucidated using a total internal reflection fluorescence microscope (TIRF). The TIRF observation was started at 1 hour after the addition of lentinan, and the number of the membrane-TNFR1 that appeared or disappeared for 15 min was counted.

Results: In the observation using CLFM, it was demonstrated that the fusion protein of GFP and TNFR1 removed intracellular domain (truncated TNFR1-GFP) was expressed in Caco-2 cell membrane, although full-length TNFR1-GFP was not detected on the membrane. The expression level of the truncated TNFR1-GFP on the cell membrane decreased when Caco-2 cells were treated with lentinan. Furthermore, it made clear in TIRF observation that the number of TNFR1 appeared on cell membrane decreased by lentinan treatment, whereas that of TNFR1 disappeared from the membrane was nearly unchanged.

Conclusion: It was ascertained that lentinan suppressed the expression of TNFR1 at the surface of cell membrane by inhibition of transportation of TNFR1 to the cell surface.

GARLIC-DERIVED S-ALLYLMERCAPTOCYSTEINE AMELIORATES THE OBESITY INDUCED BONE LOSS

Lu Zhang[1], Zhengyun Xia[2], George L. Tipoe[2], Willian Weijia Lu[1]

[1]Department of Orthopaedics and Traumatology, [2]School of Biomedical Sciences, Li Ka Shing Faculty of Medicine, The University of Hong Kong, Hong Kong SAR, China

Keywords: garlic, exercise, obesity, bone, osteoporosis

Background: Osteoporosis is a problem associated with elderly people that may induce fracture and chronic pain. Associated with the development of osteoporosis, there is an increase of fat content in bone marrow for elderly people. Studies have also indicated that the risk of osteoporosis increases for people of overweight and obesity. Since the bone generating cell, osteoblast, and the adipocyte share the same precursor, it was hypothesized that the bone volume might be maintained from a balance of adipogenesis and osteoblastogenesis. Previous study in our group indicated that *in vivo* administration of garlic-derived S-allylmercaptocysteine (SAMC) (200 mg/kg, *ip*, three times a week) significantly decreased adipocyte content in liver with non-alcoholic fatty liver disease (NAFLD) which was induced by high fat diet (Xiao et al., 2013). At the same time SAMC also down-regulated the expressions of cytokines, NF-κB and AP-1 in the animal liver. In recent experiments, our group also observed that daily endurance exercise provided a similar hepato-protective effect.

Objective: For a better understanding of the relationship of bone marrow adipocyte and osteoporosis, we investigated the effect of SAMC and endurance exercise to the bone metabolism with or without intake of high fat diet.

Methods: Female Sprague Dawley rats (180-200g) were fed with standard chow or a diet comprising highly unsaturated fat diet

(30% fish oil and other supplements) for 12 weeks. Animals eating standard chow or high fat diet were subjected to exercise on a rota wheel 30 min/day from 9th to 12th week or given intraperitoneal injection of 200 mg/kg SAMC three times per week. After euthanasia, lower limbs bones were collected for MicroCT, mechanical and histological analysis. Blood and liver samples of rats were also collected for histological and biochemical analysis.

Results: High fat diet decreased the bone mineral density (BMD) of rat tibiae proximal metaphysis trabecular bone by 0.97 standard deviation (p <0.05) which was not reversed by SAMC injection or exercise. SAMC and exercise increased the cortical bone volume for diaphysis of both femur and tibiae in animal both taking standard chow and high fat diet. Mechanical strength (maximum bending load, stiffness) in both femur and tibiae were also improved after SAMC injection or exercise even under high fat diet.

Conclusion: SAMC intake and endurance exercise could be beneficial for bone health.

ASSESSMENT OF SERUM ADIPONECTIN, LEPTIN AND SPECIFIC IGE LEVELS IN CHILDREN WITH FOOD ALLERGY

Mahshid Sirjani[1], Raheleh Shokouhi Shoormasti[1], Maryam Ayazi[1], Behnoosh Tayebi[1], Nazanin Khodayari Namini[1], Nastaran Sabetkish[1], Zahra Pourpak[1]

[1]Immunology, Asthma and Allergy Research Institute, Tehran University of Medical Sciences, Tehran, Iran.

Keywords: Leptin, adiponectin, immunoglobulin E, food allergy

Background: There is growing evidence for an association between adipokines and allergic diseases in adults. However, few studies have investigated the relationship between adipokines and food allergy especially in children.

Objective: To assess the relationship between specific immunoglobulin E (IgE) and two key adipokines -leptin, adiponectin- in children with food allergy compared to aged-sex matched healthy controls.

Methods: Forty patients with definite diagnosis of food allergy (group I) referred from December 2014 - April 2016 to Immunology, Asthma and Allergy Research Institute, were enrolled in this pilot study. Definite diagnosis was made based on history of allergic reaction to food and a positive food-specific IgE. The control group (group II) included 30 children with no evidence of allergic symptoms, who were referred for minor surgical procedures to Urology Department of Children Medical Center Hospital. Demographic and clinical characteristics of subjects were recorded using a data gathering form and informed written consent was obtained of both groups. Subjects in group I and II were age-and gender-matched. After drawing blood samples of all subjects and serum separation, leptin and adiponectin levels were measured by ELISA method. Moreover, specific IgE was measured for eight most common food allergens by immunoblot method in all participants. Regarding the association of adiponectin and leptin with body weight, Weight-for-age and body mass index (BMI)-for-age percentiles were used as growth index for subjects under and above 2 years old, respectively.

Results: The results of this study revealed that there was no significant difference in gender and age between study groups ($p > 0.05$). The median age of participants in group I and II was 18.5 (Q1=8, Q3=42) and 23.5 (Q1=18, Q3=28) months, respectively. Cesarean section rate was respectively 64.9% and 16.7% in group I and II, which showed a significant difference($p<0.001$). In addition, a significant difference was detected between group I and II in birth weight (Mean ± SD) (3.23±0.45 vs. 3.67±0.35 kg, $p<0.001$) and birth length (Mean ± SD) (0.49±0.02 vs. 0.51±0.01 meter, $p=0.002$). Serum levels of adiponectin were significantly higher in patients group compared to controls (Mean ± SD) (24.11±12.14 vs. 10.67±12.23 µg/ml $p<0.001$). No statistically significant difference was detected in serum leptin concentrations between study groups ($p =0.92$). There was a significant inverse relationship between age and adiponectin levels in group I ($p = 0.002$, $r = - 0.479$) and group II ($p =0.04$, $r= - 0.365$). However, the results were more significant in group I. In spite of a positive correlation between age and leptin level in group I, the difference was not statistically significant ($P = 0.053$, $r = 0.308$). Based on specific IgE levels the most common allergens in patient group were wheat (52.5%), hazelnut (52.5%), cow's milk (50%), and egg white (30%). According to growth rate indices, neither patient group nor control group were overweight or obese.

Conclusions: The results of this study suggest that, adiponectin levels were statistically higher in patient group, which may show pivotal link of adiponectin with food allergy. Whereas leptin does not seem to be related to food allergy. Considering the subjects' growth indices, these findings are probably unlikely to be affected by obesity as a confounding factor. A research project with a larger sample size has been designed and is currently carried out to further investigate and confirm the results of this pilot study.

OLEACEIN – A NEW APPROACH TO THE PREVENTION OF HUMAN CAROTID PLAQUE DESTABILIZATION

Agnieszka Filipek[1], Monika E. Czerwińska[1], Anna K. Kiss[1], Jerzy A. Polański[2] and Marek Naruszewicz[1]

[1]Department of Pharmacognosy and Molecular Basis of Phytotherapy, Medical University of Warsaw, Banacha 1, 02-097 Warsaw, Poland; [2]2nd Chair and Department of General, Vascular and Oncologic Surgery, Medical University of Warsaw, Żwirki i Wigury 61, 02-091 Warsaw, Poland

Keywords: oleacein, carotid plaque, plaque destabilization, atherosclerosis

Background: Many studies have shown that interplaque hemorrhage is a predisposing factor in destabilization of carotid plaque. Our recent results [Phytomedicine 22 (2015) 1255–1261] suggested that oleacein (3,4-DHPEA-EDA), a secoiridod isolated from leaves of *Ligustrum vulgare* L., together with haemoglobin and haptoglobin complex may change macrophage phenotype from pro-inflamatory M-1 to anti-inflamatory M-2. This effect was related to increased expression of CD 163 and IL-10 receptor. Since oleacein strongly interacts with red blood cells proteins, it is also likely to be present in atherosclerotic plaque during hemorrhage.

Objective: This study was to investigate effects of oleacein on carotid plague instability markers *ex vivo*. We have measured specific markers released from necrotic cells and activated macrophages, as well as foam cells present in carotid plaque.

Methods: Carotid plaques were collected immediately after the endarterectomy of 20 hypertensive patients (11 women and 9 men)

with transient ischemic attacks. Matching pieces of each plaque were incubated with oleacein in the concentration range 5-20 µM for 24 h in the presence of LPS (1 µg/ml), which is a factor inducing a destabilization.

Oleacein, oleuropein, oleocanthal, hydroxytyrosol and tyrosol were isolated from *Ligustrum vulgare* L. leaves. The purity of compounds was confirmed by HPLC-DAD-MS^n method. High-mobility group protein B1 (HMGB1), metalloproteinase 9 (MMP-9), MMP-9/ neutrophil gelatinase-associated lipocalin complex (MMP-9/NGAL), tissue factor (TF) and interleukin-10 (IL-10), as well as heme oxygenase (HO-1) secretion from activated plaques was measured by enzyme-linked immunosorbent assay (ELISA).

Results: Oleacein at the concentrations of 10 and 20 µM significantly ($p<0.001$) decreased secretion from the treated plaques: HMGB1 (up 90%), MMP-9 (up to 80%), MMP-9/NGAL complex (up to 80%) and TF (more than 90%), as compared to control. At the same time IL-10 and HO-1 release increased by more than 80% ($p<0.001$). Such properties have not been demonstrated for other polyphenols, i.e. oleuropein, oleocanthal, hydroxytyrosol and tyrosol.

Conclusion: Our results indicate that oleacein possess ability to attenuate the destabilization process of carotid plaque probably by increased removal of red blood cells – derived hemoglobin through macrophages CD163 receptor. Thus, it may be assumed that oleacein as a food supplement for a special medical purpose may be useful in the primary prevention of cerebral ischaemia and stroke.

IMPACT OF CASEIN NON-PHOSPHOPEPTIDES ON SARCOPENIA USING CT SCANNING TECHNOLOGY

Na Zhang [1], Yan-Guo Shi [1], Qing-Qi Guo [2], Chang-Hui Guo[1]

[1]Key Laboratory of Food Science and Engineering of Heilongjiang Province, Harbin University of Commerce, 36# No.138, TongDa Street, DaoLi District, Harbin 150076, P R China; [2]Forestry School, Northeast Forestry University, No.26, HeXing Street, XiangFang District, Harbin 150040, P R China

Keywords: Casein non-phosphopeptide; Sarcopenia; whey protein; CT scanning

Background: About 1%~2% people suffer from sarcopenia after the age of 50 and the percent affected reaches more than 50% after the age of 80. Sarcopenia could lead to weakened strength, digressive balance movement ability, diabetes, arthritis, osteoporosis and heart disease. Some scientists used the leucine-rich lactalbumin to resist sarcopenia. However, the cost of lactalbumin is very high.

Objective: To determine the anti-sarcopenia effect of Casein non-phosphopeptide (CNPP), which is a byproduct formed during casein phosphopeptide (CPP) preparation.

Methods: CNPP was fed to 64 rats (32-weeks-old). The trunk and lower limb muscle group, lumbar muscle group, back muscle group, beta scapular muscle group, left upper limb muscles root group, right upper limb axillary fat of rats were classified into resistive exercise group (REG) and free exercise group (FEG), which was determined by using transverse spiral CT scanning at fedding 0, 15, 25, 35, 50 days, respectively. The glucose level, growth hormone content, insulin level and testosterone content of rats was analyzed by kit method, respectively. Lactalbumin was used as a contrast.

Results: The results showed that the cross-sectional area growth rate of the trunk and lower limb muscle group, the back muscle group and beta scapular muscle group of FEG rats, which were fed CNPP and lactalbumin increased. The cross-sectional area growth rates of the back muscles, beta scapular muscle group of REG rats, which were fed CNPP or lactalbumin also increased. However, the cross-sectional area growth rates of CNPP feeding groups were less than the lactalbumin feeding group. The testosterone level, content of growth hormone and insulin level in the blood of the REG and FEG rats of CNPP feeding groups and the lactalbumin feeding groups all increased. However, the content of growth hormone in the blood of the REG and FEG rats of the CNPP feeding groups were higher than that of the lactalbumin feeding groups. The testosterone level, insulin level in the REG and FEG rats, which were fed CNPP were lower than that of in lactalbumin feeding group.

Conclusion: Our study demonstrated that the leucine-rich CNPP could stimulate the synthesis of some muscle, insulin level, content of growth hormone, and testosterone level.

KEY ENZYME INHIBITORY PROPERTIES RELATED TO SOME NON-COMMUNICABLE DISEASES FROM DEFATTED RICE BRAN PROTEIN ISOLATE AND PROTEIN HYDROLYSATES

Natchanan Yotpinta[1], Nattapol Tungsuphoom[1], Nattira On-nom[1], Yuraporn Sahasakul[1], Chatrapa Hudthagosol[2], Promluck Somboonpanyakul[2], Suwimol Sapwarobol[3] and Uthaiwan Suttisansanee[1]

[1]Institute of Nutrition, Mahidol University, Nakhon Pathom, 73170, Thailand; [2]Department of Nutrition, Faculty of Public Health, Mahidol University, Bangkok, 10400, Thailand; [3]Department of Nutrition and Dietetics, Faculty of Allied Health Sciences, Chulalongkorn University, Bangkok, 10330, Thailand

Keywords: Defatted rice bran protein, protein isolate, protein hydrolysates, non-communicable diseases

Background: Defatted rice bran (DRB) powder is a major co-product from rice bran oil industry. DRB powder contains several useful nutrients such as dietary fiber, iron, vitamin B1 and B3. Especially, it contains 12-15% protein content. Thus, DRB is a good source of inexpensive, high quality protein. Protease digested rice bran proteins were previously reported to exhibit various pharmacological properties such as anti-diabetic, anti-dyslipidemic and anti- hypertensive effects. Therefore, DRB powder might be a good source for protein isolates and protein hydrolysates with potential health properties that function against some non-communicable diseases.

Objective: To prepare the DRB protein isolate (DRBPI) by acid-base precipitation and DRB protein hydrolysates (DRBPH) by enzymatic hydrolysis to investigate functional (degree of hydrolysis (DH), solubility and amino acid profile) and biochemical properties (antioxidants activity and key enzyme inhibitory properties against obesity (lipase), diabetes (α-amylase and α-glucosidase), hypertension (angiotensin-converting enzyme, ACE) and Alzheimer's disease (acetylcholinesterase (AChE) and butyrylcholinesterase (BChE)).

Methods: DRBPI was optimally isolated from DRB powder in basic buffer (pH 12) at 50-55°C for 1 hour. DRBPI was then precipitated in acidic buffer (pH 4) and re-solubilized in buffer (pH 8). DRBPI was hydrolyzed by alcalase, flavozyme and protamex with optimum conditions including hydrolysis time of 180 minutes and enzyme-to-substrate ratio of 2%. Alcalase was optimally functioned at temperature of 55°C in buffer pH 9, while flavozyme and protamex preferred a working temperature of 50°C in buffer pH 6 and pH 7, respectively. DRBPH and DRBPI were then investigated regarding antioxidant activities (ferric reducing antioxidant power (FRAP) and oxygen radical absorbance capacity (ORAC) assays) and key enzyme inhibitory properties (lipase, α-amylase, α-glucosidase, ACE, AChE and BChE.

Results: As results, amino acid profile of DRBPI was rich in Glu, Tyr, Asp and His, while Met was the limiting amino acid. Solubility of DRBPI was elevated with increasing pH (higher than isoelectric point or pH 4), and the highest solubility was found at pH 8. Likewise, solubility of DRBPH was optimized at pH 8. The highest degree of hydrolysis (DH) values for each DRBPH was 14.29% for alcalase, 12.01% for flavozyme and 6.03% for protamex. Antioxidant activities of DRBPH were higher than those of DRBPI with alcalase digested DRBPH exhibiting the highest antioxidant activity (1403.81 μmol TE/g by ORAC assay). However, the antioxidant activities as being measured by FRAP assay suggested that DRBPI was a better source of antioxidants than DRBPH. The results from enzyme inhibitory properties including anti-α-glucosidase, anti-ACE and anti-BChE activities suggested that DRBPH exhibited significantly higher anti-enzyme activities than those of DRBPI. Anti-α-amylase and anti-lipase activities of DRBPI were, on the other hand, higher than those of DRBPH. Nevertheless, anti-AChE activities were not detected for all samples.

Conclusion: DRBPH is possibly a rich source of anti-hypertensive and anti-Alzheimer's disease agents, while DRBPI provides potential anti-obesity and anti-diabetic agents. These results can provide alternative prevention of these non-communicable diseases as well as potential development of functional ingredients, functional food products and nutraceuticals. Moreover, this research could provide the suitable enzyme conditions for protein hydrolysate preparation from DRB for industrial food manufacturing.

NUTRITIONAL EVALUATION, BIOACCUMULATION AND TOXICOLOGICAL ASSESSMENT OF HEAVY METALS IN EDIBLE FRUITS OF *FICUS SUR FORSSK (MORACEAE)*

Olumuyiwa O. Ogunlaja[1], Roshila Moodley[1], Himansu Baijnath[2] and Sreekanth Jonnalagadda[1]

[1]Natural Product Research Laboratory, School of Chemistry and Physics, University of KwaZulu-Natal, Westville, 4000 Durban, South Africa. [2]School of Life Sciences, University of KwaZulu-Natal, Westville, 4000 Durban, South Africa

Keywords: Elemental distribution, nutrition, health, toxicity, soil quality

Background: *Ficus sur* (Moraceae) is an indigenous medicinal plant with a wide distribution in Africa. It is known as Umkhiwane by the Zulu people and serves as an immediate source of food both to animals and humans, hence playing a key role in their everyday survival, especially during times of famine. Previous study reveals the presence of pharmacologically active triterpenoids.

Objective: To investigate the nutritional and health potential of an indigenous plant, *F. sur Forssk* fruits to meet domestic food demands and reduce food insecurity in KwaZulu-Natal, South Africa. The proximate composition, phytocompounds and concentrations of metals in the edible fruits and the growth soil collected from eight different sites in KwaZulu-Natal were determined in order to assess for nutritional value and the impact of soil quality on elemental uptake.

Methods: The proximate composition and concentrations of metals in the edible fruits collected from eight different sites in

KwaZulu-Natal were determined by the Association of Official Analytical Chemists (AOAC) method to assess for nutritional value and the concentrations of metals in the growth soil was determined to evaluate the impact of soil quality on elemental uptake.

Results: The fruits contained high levels of moisture ($88.8 \pm 0.2\%$) and carbohydrates ($65.6 \pm 0.03\%$). The fruits also contained $5.2 \pm 0.1\%$ of protein, $4.7 \pm 0.2\%$ of fat, $7.7 \pm 0.02\%$ of crude fibre and $17.67 \pm 1.3\%$ of ash. The concentrations of elements in the fruits were found to be in decreasing order of Ca > Mg > Fe > Zn > Cu > Mn > Se with low levels of toxic metals (As, Cd, Co and Pb). Calcium concentrations in fruits ranged from 2270 to 7746 $\mu g \ g^{-1}$ with bioaccumulation factor (BAF) between 0.6 and 6.0 indicating the tendency of the plant to accumulate this metal. The fruit also tended to accumulate Mg producing BAFs (Exchangeable) between 16.9 and 91.5 even though, Mg mobility was low (0.4 to 29.2%). Consumption of 20.0 g of *F. sur* fruits may contribute between 8.4 -11.0% and 9.0-9.2% towards the Recommended Dietary Allowance (RDA) for Ca and Mg respectively. In addition, two pharmacologically active triterpenoids (β-sitosterol and lupeol) with documented anti-inflammatory activity and cholesterol-lowering effect were isolated from the fruit respectively. The fruit also contains a strong antioxidant, (+)-catechin, which has been shown to have cardio-protective benefits by its profibrinolytic effect on cultured human coronary artery endothelial cells.

Conclusion: Data from this study indicates that the fruits can serve as an immediate and alternative source of energy due to high level of carbohydrates. This study shows that the consumption of the fruits of *F. sur* can help to prevent chronic non-communicable diseases and contribute positively to the nutritional needs and health of rural communities in South Africa for most essential nutrients without posing the risk of adverse health effects.

ANTIOXIDANT AND CYTOTOXICITY ACTIVITIES OF CRUDE EXTRACTS AND COMPOUNDS FROM LEAVES AND STEM BARK OF *FICUS BURTT-DAVYI*

Olumuyiwa O. Ogunlaja [1], Roshila Moodley [1], Himansu Baijnath [2], Moganaveli Singh[3] and Sreekanth Jonnalagadda [1]

[1] Natural Product Research Laboratory, School of Chemistry and Physics, University of KwaZulu-Natal, Westville, 4000 Durban, South Africa. [2] School of Life Sciences, University of KwaZulu-Natal, Westville, 4000 Durban, South Africa. [3] Non-viral Gene delivery Laboratory, School of Biochemistry, University of KwaZulu-Natal, Westville, 4000 Durban, South Africa

Keywords: *Ficus burtt-davyi*, phaeophytin, triterpenes, flavonoids, antioxidants, cytotoxicity

Background: *Ficus burtt-davyi*, is an endemic species of South Africa, belonging to the genus Ficus, with over 850 species. Ficus (Moraceae) is one of the oldest, most successful, but understudied genera in modern pharmacognosy with extensive distribution of secondary metabolites such as triterpeniods, phenolics, flavonoids, alkaloids, coumarins and sterols. Many species of the genus Ficus have shown documented biological activities. *F. burtt-davyi,* known as Uluzi by the Zulu people in KwaZulu-Natal, is highly adaptable to a wide variety of habitats and has even been known to grow on larger trees (epiphytic) as a strangler fig, as well as on rocks (epilithic) where the roots are able to split the rocks in their search for nutrients. To date, no information has been reported on the chemical composition, antioxidant and cytotoxicity activity of this plant.

Objective: To probe *F. burtt-davyi* as a possible source of secondary metabolites, we phytochemically investigated leaves and stem bark and assessed the in-vitro antioxidant activity, as well the cytotoxicity activity of extracts and isolated compounds using human cancer cell lines.

Methods: Isolated compounds were characterized using NMR spectroscopy and by comparison with literature values. Extracts from the leaves, stem bark and isolated compounds were investigated for their antioxidant activity using 1, 1-diphenyl-2-picryl hydrazyl (DPPH) free radical scavenging, Ferric reducing power (FRAP) and Hydrogen peroxide-scavenging assays. Cytotoxicity investigation was also carried out by using the mitochondrial dependent reduction of yellow MTT to purple formazan against the human breast carcinoma (MCF-7) and colorectal adenocarcinoma (Caco-2) cell lines, with 5- fluorouracil (5-FU) as positive control.

Results: In vitro antioxidant study of methanol extracts of leaves and stem bark, (+)-catechin and phaeophytin **a** using 1,1-diphenyl-1-picrylhydrazyl (DPPH) free radical scavenging assay, ferric reducing antioxidant power (FRAP) assay and hydrogen peroxide (H_2O_2) assay showed significantly higher ($p< 0.05$) antioxidant activity for the methanol extract of the stem bark than the leaves, with IC_{50} values of 58.28 ± 5.05 for DPPH, 46.09 ± 0.06 for FRAP and 151.03 ± 1.60 $\mu g\ mL^{-1}$ for H_2O_2. The methanol extract from the stem bark was significantly cytotoxic (MTT assay) to MCF-7 and Caco-2 cell lines ($p < 0.05$) in a concentration-dependent manner with cell viability inhibition of 80.0 and 91.0 % at concentration of 1 and 25 $\mu g\ mL^{-1}$ respectively.

Conclusion: Phytochemical analysis of leaves and stem bark yielded five triterpenes (lupeol, lupeol acetate, β-sitosterol, stigmasterol and campesterol), one carotenoid (lutein), a phaeophytin (phaeophytin **a**) and one flavonoid (+)-catechin). The data from this study suggests that *F. burtt-davyi* possessed moderate to good anti-oxidative activity and can be used as a potential alternative medicine for oxidative stress related non-communicable chronic diseases. The phytochemical and cytotoxic results from our study also indicated that (+)-catechin and lupeol, the most abundant bioactive compound in the stem bark are responsible for the synergetic cytotoxic effect of this extract against breast and colorectal adenocarcinoma cell lines.

IMPROVEMENT OF ABNORMAL FAT METABOLISM BY SULFORAPHANE THROUGH THE ENDOPLASMIC RETICULUM STRESS IN HEPATOCYTES

Sicong Tian and Yujuan Shan

School of Chemistry and Chemical Engineering, Harbin Institute of Technology, Harbin, 150090, China

Keywords: sulforaphane, Non-alcoholic fatty liver, ER stress

Background: Sulforaphane (SFN), which is existed as precursors of glucosinolates (GS) in cruciferous vegetables has been reported to regulate lipid metabolism. Endoplasmic reticulum stress(ERS), has been identified as one of the key mechanisms in process of lipid accumulation, say triglycerides (TG) and cholesterol(TC), in non-alcoholic fatty liver disease (NAFLD). Inositol-requiring enzyme-1(IRE1), ER stress sensor, activated by unfolded proteins by releasing from glucose-regulated protein(GRP78), splices X-box-binding protein-1 (XBP1) transcripts to form a transcription factor to activate lipogenesis while inhibit gluconeogenesis through sterol regulatory element-binding proteins (SREBP1) which regulate lipogenic enzymes including acetyl-CoA carboxylase 1 (ACC1), fatty acid synthase (FAS), and stearoyl-CoA desaturase 1 (SCD1). We previously found SFN was able to inhibit GRP78 caused by homocysteine and regulate SREBP1 in alcohol-induced injury rats.

Objectives: The goal is to investigate the protection mechanism of SFN in NAFLD by SREBP-1 activation via ERS in hepatocytes.

Methods: The hepatocytes, the HHL-5 cells, was incubated with medium (DMEM/F12 1:1) containing 10% fetal bovine serum. Cultured cells were pre-protected by SFN in dose- and time-effect relationship, then exposed to 300 μmol/L FFAs (oleic acid: palmitic acid, 1:2). To study whether SFN can decrease lipid contents in HHL-5, oil red O was used to stain intracellular lipids droplets. TG and TC levels, as well as aspartate aminotransferase (AST) and alanine aminotransferase(ALT) activity were measured using assay kit. Further, transmission electron microscopy was used to observe endoplasmic reticulum structure change under FFAs and recovery by SFN. Moreover, to understand the molecular mechanism of SFN improving the abnormal fat metabolism, we studied the ER transcription regulatory protein XBP1, GRP78 expression as well as SREBP 1and ACC1, FAS, SCD1 by RT-PCR; after total cell protein being obtained, XBP1 and SREBP1 were analyzed by western blot.

Results: 300 μmol/L FFAs significantly increased the number of lipid droplets and TC & TG levels in HHL-5 cells compared with control group, so as the ALT and AST activity ($P<0.01$). However, compared with positive control group TG and TC levels decreased significantly after pre-protection of SFN in dose- and time-effect relationship ($P < 0.01$). Being stimulated by FAAs caused endoplasmic reticulum expansion in HHL-5 cells, which suggested endoplasmic reticulum dysfunction, while for SFN protection group, endoplasmic reticulum expansion obviously improved. RT-PCR detection of XBP1, GRP78, SREBP 1, ACC1, FAS, SCD1mRNA expression showed that FAAs induced HHL-5 cells to express more quantity of XBP1, GRP78 and SREBP1 mRNA than control group by approximately 15%, 18%, and 23%, respectively. Meanwhile, expression quantity of ACC1, FAS mRNA also increased while SCD1 remained stable. SFN in dose- and time-effect relationship pro-protect cells reduced mRNA expression quantity of XBP1, GRP78,SREBP1 and synthesis of lipids related enzymes except SCD1. Compared with an increase of protein expressions of XBP1 and SREBP1 under the inducer, SFN down-regulated the expression in dose- and time-effect relationship.

Conclusion: Taken together, the present findings suggest the molecular biological mechanism of SFN reducing disorders of lipid metabolism caused by oleic acid/palmitic acid in HHL-5 cells through inhibiting ERS.

INDUSTRIAL DEFATTED RICE BRAN POWDER: A POTENT THERAPEUTIC AGENT FOR THE PREVENTION AND TREATMENT OF CERTAIN CHRONIC DISEASES

Suwapat Kittibunchakul[1], Chatrapa Hudthagosol[2], Promluck Somboonpanyakul[2], Suwimol Sapwarobol[3], and Uthaiwan Suttisansanee[1]

[1]Institute of Nutrition, Mahidol University, Nakhon Pathom, 73170, Thailand; [2]Department of Nutrition, Faculty of Public Health, Mahidol University, Bangkok, 10400, Thailand; [3]Department of Nutrition and Dietetics, Faculty of Allied Health Sciences, Chulalongkorn University, Bangkok, 10330, Thailand

Keywords: Defatted rice bran, chronic disease, enzyme inhibitory property

Background: At present, green medicine from plants and natural products are of interest to improve health and prevent some non-communicable diseases due to its consumption safety with less side effects comparing to those of synthetic drugs. Likewise, therapeutic roles of defatted rice bran (DRB) powder, which is the co-product derived from rice bran oil production, has currently been called to attention in order to obtain the full benefit of phytochemicals in rice bran. Interestingly, previous research had shown that DRB still contains several types of antioxidants and bioactive compounds with possible inhibitory effects on disease-related enzymes.

Objective: To provide supportive evidence for extending the utilization of DRB powder, we explored antioxidant activities, anti-aging properties and potential suppression of some chronic disorders including obesity, diabetes, Alzheimer's disease and hypertension from DRB extract. Phenolics including phenolic acids and flavonoids remaining in DRB were, as well, identified and quantified.

Methods: Commercial DRB powders with the particle size of 140 and 200 meshes provided by the manufacturer were extracted with 40% (v/v) aqueous ethanol at 30 °C in a water bath shaker for 2 h. Therapeutic potentials of the extracts were analyzed using spectrophotometric and fluorometric assays. Antioxidant activities were tested by ferric reducing antioxidant power (FRAP), 2,2-diphenyl-1-picrylhydrazyl (DPPH) radical scavenging and oxygen radical absorbance capacity (ORAC) assays, while total phenolic contents (TPCs) were analyzed by Folin-Ciocalteu reagent. The inhibitions of glycation reaction induced by glucose and methylglyoxal were employed for investigating anti-aging property. Besides, inhibitory potentials toward obesity (lipase), diabetes (α-amylase and α-glucosidase), Alzheimer's disease (acetylcholinesterase; AChE and butyrylcholinesterase; BChE) and hypertension (angiotensin converting enzyme; ACE) were explored based on the inhibitory reaction against key enzymes that control these diseases. Effects of particle size on the activities of DRB were, as well, observed. Phenolic acids and flavonoids in DRB were identified and quantified using a high performance liquid chromatography (HPLC).

Results: Size reduction did not clearly improve inhibitory potentials of DRB. However, DRB with a smaller particle size (200-mesh) tended to provide slightly higher activities in comparison to DRB with a larger particle size (140-mesh). Antioxidant activities of DRB powders were 127.07-148.87, 0.052-0.054 and 219.06-345.30 μmol TE/g as being detected by FRAP, DPPH radical scavenging and ORAC assays, respectively. Their TPCs were 14.32-15.50 mg GAE/g. The half maximal inhibitory concentration (IC_{50}) values for glucose-induced glycation were 5.48-7.56 mg/mL, and those for methylglyoxal-induced glycation were 25.24-33.92 mg/mL. DRB offered inhibitory properties against lipase, α-amylase, α-glucosidase, AChE and BChE with the proximate inhibitions of 12, 21, 5, 20 and 88% (at concentration of 50 mg/mL), respectively. Interestingly, DRB exhibited strong inhibition toward ACE (approximately 80% inhibitions at the concentration of 5 mg/mL). The analysis of phenolics showed that DRB (140-mesh) was predominated by ferulic acid (402.54 mg/100 g) and *p*-coumaric acid (128.59 mg/100 g). However, there were no flavonoids detected in this study.

Conclusion: The knowledge received from this research demonstrated that DRB powder possibly confers special health benefits in reducing the risk of some chronic diseases beyond providing nutritional value of dietary fibers, proteins and vitamin B. The data also support the potential of DRB for health utilizations and future commercial availability. With the refinement of manufacturing process and the further product development, DBR will be applicable as a low-cost functional ingredient and healthy supplement for human consumption and therapeutic use.

HEALTH BENEFIT, FOOD SAFETY AND PRODUCT DEVELOPMENT OF LOCAL PLANTS AT CONSERVED AREA OF PLANT GENETIC CONSERVATION PROJECT UNDER THE ROYAL INITIATIVE OF HER ROYAL HIGHNESS PRINCESS MAHA CHAKRI SIRINDHORN, KANCHANABURI PROVINCE, THAILAND

Uthaiwan Suttisansanee, Warangkana Srichamnong, Nattira On-nom, Parunya Thiyajai, Rungrat Chamchan, Kunchit Judprasong and Somsri Charoenkiatkul

Institute of Nutrition, Mahidol University, Nakhon Pathom, 73170, Thailand

Keywords: Local food plants, biochemical properties, safety, product development, healthy food

Background: Food plants from forests and local food plants are important food sources for many villagers in Thailand. The advantage of these plants includes safety for daily consumption as vegetables or as traditional medicines. This project was aimed to pursue the works of the Plant Genetic Conservation Project under the initiative of Her Royal Highness Princess Maha Chakri Sirindhorn using collaboration between researchers and communities in the area of Khuean Srinagarindra National Park, Kanchanaburi Province, Thailand.

Objective: To investigate the health benefit, food safety and product development of local plants in conserved area of Plant Genetic Conservation Project under the Royal Initiative of Her Royal Highness Princess Maha Chakri Sirindhorn, Kanchanaburi Province, Thailand

Methods: The health properties of 48 local plant foods to fight against chronic degenerative diseases including obesity (anti-lipase activity), diabetes (anti-α-glucosidase and anti-α-amylase activities), hypertension (anti-angiotensin-converting enzyme), Alzheimer's disease (anti-cholinesterase, anti-β-secretase and antioxidant activities) and ageing (anti-glycation and anti-tyrosinase activities) were screened, and the first top 20 were further investigated with the communities regarding their properties as being traditional herbal medicines. Then, the selected top 10 local food plants were examined regarding their health properties against previously mentioned non-communicable diseases through key enzyme inhibitions, plant toxins and contaminations from nature. A further research on the development of food products was conducted with the community.

Results: The selected top 10 local food plants with high traditional medical properties and health benefits were Kra Don (*Barringtonia acutangula* (L.) Gaertn.), Makham Pom (*Phyllanthus emblica* L.), Pak Kood (*Diplazium esculentum* (Retz.) Sw.), Kra Pee Jun (*Millettia brandisiana* Kurz), Ka Pah (*Alpinia malaccensis* (Burm.)Roscoe.), Phlai (*Zingiber cassumunar* Roxb.), Ta Kuek (*Albiziz Lebbeck* (L.) Benth), Wan Pro (*Kaempferia roscoeana* Wall.), Kra Chai Pran (*Zingiber citriodorum* J. Mood & T. Theleide) and Mara Pah (*Momordica charantia* L.). Overall, it was found that Kra Don exhibited the highest health properties, while Mara Pah exhibited the least. The highest amount of saponin was found in Kra Don, while Kra Chai Pran contained the highest level of total alkaloid. Lectin was found in trace amount, and none was detected in Kra Don. Heavy metals including lead and cadmium were detected in all plant samples, while total arsenic was not found in Kra Pee Jun, Ta Kuek and Makham Pom. Overall, all metals were below the standard limit. Even though these food plants contained phytotoxins and heavy metals, the effect on human health would be neglectable if avoiding over-consumption. From these data along with traditional knowledge on consumption and intellectual preparation of indigenous plants, sour vegetable curry (Geang-Som-Ta-Kuek) and country style red curry (Geang-Pa-Kra-Chai-Pran) had been selected and reformulated by reducing sodium content (8 and 40%, respectively). Geang-Som-Ta-Kuek was low in energy and fat, while Geang-Pa-Kra-Chai-Pran contained medium energy and fat. Moreover, both recipes were source of fiber and contained high total phenolics and antioxidant activities. Besides, chili paste with herbal plants (Wan Prao, Kra Chai Pran, Ka Pah and Phlai) and grilled fish was developed as healthy food product with 92% acceptance of consumers. In order to create awareness of local resource preservation to maintain food supply, knowledge and technology on health benefits, food safety and product development from local plant foods were transferred back to the locals who live around Khuean Srinagarindra National Park, Kanchanaburi Province, Thailand with positive response.

Conclusion: This research presents the potential of local plants in terms of health benefits, safety for household consumption and development of local products. This research can be a prototype to develop other local foods with suitable taste and health benefits for visitors or tourists. The research could support local job opportunity and increase overall local income. Moreover, this research also supported local awareness to maintain food supply in the community.

THE NATURAL PROBIOTIC MINE: KEFIR GRAINS

Zeynep Banu Guzel-Seydim, Sevgi Atılgan, Tugba Kok Tas, A. Can Seydim

Suleyman Demirel University Faculty of Engineering Department of Food Engineering Isparta 32260 Turkey

Keywords: kefir grains, probiotic, fermented foods, prebiotic, health attributes, *Lactobacillus kefiranfaciens*, *Lactobacillus kefiri*

Background: The tribes in the Northern Caucasus mountain region first described Kefir grains. Kefir is produced by fermentative activity of "kefir grains" which contain a diverse range of inherent lactic acid bacteria, yeast, and sometimes acetic acid bacteria in a polysaccharide matrix of semi-hard granules. When kefir grains are added to milk and incubated for approximately 22 h at 25°C, microorganisms in the grains continue to proliferate in milk with the production of the lactic acid and other flavor compounds causing physicochemical changes. The resultant product, kefir, is a self-carbonated, refreshing fermented drink which has a unique flavor due to a mixture of lactic acid, carbon dioxide, acetaldehyde, acetoin, slight alcohol, and other fermentation flavor products. One feature of kefir that differs from other fermented milk products is that kefir grains are recovered after fermentation. The biomass of kefir grains slowly increases during the process of kefir fermentation. Resultant kefir is a natural source of probiotics and have significant health attributes.

Objective: The aim of this review manuscript is to provide significant information on kefir grains as a probiotic mine and to report the recent studies on the functional properties of kefir.

Methods: Kefir grain keeps its mystery, because it cannot be produced without the presence of single grain as a seed. The health attributes of kefir have been extensively studied rather than technological properties of kefir. In this review, the recent research papers were investigated.

Results: The microflora embedded in the grain structure consists of *Lactobacillus kefir*, *L. kefiranofaciens*, *L. kefirgranum*, *L. acidophilus*, *L. helveticus*, *L. plantarum*, *L. brevis*, *L. casei*, *L. rhamnossus*, *L. bulgaricus*, *L. fermentum*, *L. gasseri*, *Lactococcus lactis* subsp. *lactis*, *Lc. lactis* subsp. *lactis* biovar. *diacetylactis*, *Lc. lactis* subsp. *cremoris*, *Streptococcus thermophilus*, *Bifidobacterium* spp. *Acetobacter* ssp., *Saccharomyces cerevisiae*, *Kluyveromyces lactis* and *Kluyveromyces marxianus*. Kefir grain resembles the probiotic supplementation with its protective mainly polysaccharide outer part. Kefir is known to have positive effects on health, especially digestive system, intestinal health, immune system and neural system because of its highly probiotic microflora and metabolites such as exopolysaccharides (kefiran), organic acids, free fatty acids, bacteriocins, bioactive peptides and enzymes. Anticarcinogenic properties of kefir have been also widely discussed. Regular consumption of natural fermented dairy products especially kefir should be included in a functional diet.

Conclusion: Kefir is a distinctive fermented dairy product due to the unique, multi-species natural kefir grains used as the starter culture during the product manufacture. The microbiological and chemical composition of kefir provides a complex probiotic effect due to the inherent lactic acid bacteria and yeast. The metabolic substances produced during fermentation have proven nutraceutical activities. Such positive health properties lend credence to the view that kefir is a valuable food and warrants further laboratory and clinical study.

PART 13

Current Research and Development of New Functional Food Products

A NOVEL PHYTO-OXYLIPIN CX CONFERS ACUTE AND SYSTEMIC ANTI-INFLAMMATORY EFFECT IN THE LIVER AND SMALL INTESTINE

Amanda L Stefanson[1] and Marica Bakovic[1]

[1]Department of Human Health and Nutritional Sciences, University of Guelph, Guelph, Ontario, Canada

Keywords: Nrf2, heme oxygenase, intestine, liver, inflammation, phytochemical

Background: Nuclear factor (erythroid-derived 2)-like 2 [Nrf2] is a transcription factor responsible for the regulation of a set of anti-oxidant, anti-inflammatory and DNA protective genes by binding the anti-oxidant response element [ARE]. Heme oxygenase 1 [Hmox1] is an ARE-responsive, stress-inducible enzyme that plays an important role in resolving inflammation. Hmox1 is variable and upregulation results in decreased neutrophil infiltration of the small intestine and decreased expression of inflammatory factors.

Objective: To evaluate the effect of novel phyto-oxylipin CX on Nrf2 activation and resulting Hmox1 expression on acute intestinal and systemic inflammation.

Methods: Twelve, three-month old male C57BL/6 mice were divided into 4 groups and treated twice daily with 5 mg/kg phyto-oxylipin (CX) or sulforaphane (SF); positive (PC) and negative (NC) control groups were vehicle-treated. After seven days, mice received an intra-peritoneal injection of lipopolysaccharide (LPS; 5 mg/kg) (CX, SF, PC) or saline (NC) and were sacrificed after 4 hours. Plasma was recovered by cardiac puncture for analysis of inflammatory cytokines by multiplex ELISA; duodena were formalin-fixed, slide-mounted and H&E stained for microscopy imaging and immunohistochemistry. Small intestinal mucosa was isolated and tissues were flash frozen for gene and protein expression analysis.

Results: Hepatic Nrf2 was upregulated in all LPS-treated groups, however Nrf2 target genes showed differential responses. Hmox1 was upregulated in all groups but only reached significance for phyto-oxylipin CX group (p=0.008). Other target genes, NAD(P)H dehydrogenase quinone 1 [Nqo1] showed no treatment effect at all in the liver. H&E stained duodena tissues were was evaluated for tissue architecture and inflammatory cell infiltration. Remarkably, qualitative score analysis established that CX demonstrated less inflammatory cell infiltration than the negative control despite LPS treatments. Additionally, there was a higher crypt epithelial mitotic rate in the PC and SF groups relative to NC and CX groups (p=0.018), suggesting an increased rate of intestinal epithelial turnover that was suppressed by CX treatments.

Conclusion: Our study demonstrated that novel phyto-oxylipin CX effectively upregulates Nrf2 and Hmox1 expression in the liver. Additionally, CX showed a remarkable suppression of inflammatory cell infiltration in the duodenum despite LPS treatment, to levels below that of the saline treated control.

DISCOVERY AND IMPACT OF ZINC ON HUMAN HEALTH: BIO-MARKERS OF ZINC DEFICIENCY

Ananda S. Prasad

Wayne State University School of Medicine, Dept. of Oncology, and Karmanos Cancer Center, Detroit, Michigan, USA

Keywords: zinc, immunity, growth, thymulin, IL-2

Background: Zinc deficiency in human was recognized for the first time in 1963 and RDA for zinc was established by US National Academy of Sciences in 1974. The present WHO estimate is that nearly 2 billion subjects living in the developing world may have a zinc deficiency. The major adverse clinical effects of zinc deficiency are growth retardation, decreased cell-mediated immunity, impairment of cognitive functions, increased oxidative stress and upregulation of inflammatory cytokines. Our studies in 1963 established for the first time that zinc was essential for human health and that its deficiency occurred in the Middle East. This is due to high phytate content of their diet, which renders zinc unavailable for absorption. Conditioned deficiency of zinc has now been reported in many diseases, such as cirrhosis of the liver, chronic renal disease, malabsorption syndrome, chronic alcoholism, sickle cell disease, and other chronic diseases including malignancies.

The major clinical effects of zinc deficiency in humans include severe growth retardation, hypogonadism, cell-mediated immune dysfunction, increased oxidative stress, up-regulation of inflammatory cytokines generation, problem with healing and cognitive functions impairment.

We now know of over 300 enzymes that are zinc dependent and over two-thousand transcription factors require zinc for their functions. Zinc is now known to be a second messenger for immune cells. Zinc is essential for cell-mediated immunity, and zinc is both an antioxidant and anti-inflammatory agent. The intracellular zinc level is tightly controlled and for its homeostasis, we now know that there are 14 ZIP and 10 ZNT transporters.

Therapeutic impact of zinc on human health: Therapeutic impact of zinc on human health is also overwhelming. Zinc is being used for the treatment of acute diarrhea in infants and children in developing countries globally and this has resulted in saving millions of lives. Zinc is now an approved drug for the treatment and maintenance therapy of a serious fatal genetic disorder Wilson's disease. According to a recent Cochrane review, zinc is the only treatment, which is effective in decreasing the incidence of infections and pain crises in patients with sickle cell disease. Zinc acetate lozenges have been shown to decrease the duration of common cold by fifty percent, provided the treatment is started within 24 h of the onset of the common cold symptoms, the solution chemistry of the zinc preparation is proper and the zinc dosages are adequate.

Age related macular degeneration (AMD) accounts for a large number of legal blindness in elderly subjects throughout the world, Age Related Eye Disease study Group (AREDS) supported by the National Eye Institute. NIH has now reported the results of their ten-year zinc supplementation study in patients with AMD. Zinc was effective in decreasing the incidences of blindness and progression of AMD in elderly subjects. Most importantly zinc supplemented subjects showed increased longevity and this was due to a decrease in the cardiovascular events. No other micronutrient has shown this dramatic effect on decreasing the mortality in the elderly.

Our placebo-controlled zinc supplementation trial in the elderly has shown that zinc supplementation decreased the incidence of infections by 66% and improved the cell-mediated immunity. Also, we showed that oxidative stress markers and gene expression of inflammatory cytokines were decreased in elderly subjects who received zinc supplementation. These studies indicate that zinc supplementation to the elderly may have a preventive role in atherosclerosis.

Bio-markers of zinc deficiency: We assayed zinc in plasma, red blood cells, 24 –h urine, and hair and these were significantly decreased in comparison to the Egyptian controls of similar ages. We assayed zinc by dithizone technique. We utilized Zn^{65} to study zinc metabolism in these dwarfs. Plasma Zn^{65} turnover rate was increased and 24 h exchangeable zinc pool was decreased. We concluded from these results that the dwarfs were zinc deficient. This was the first demonstration that zinc deficiency in humans occurred.

Subsequently, in Detroit, we developed a human model that would allow us to study the effects of a mild zinc deficient state in humans and also provide us with sensitive bio-markers of zinc deficiency. We recruited adult human volunteers for induction of dietary zinc deficiency. A semi-purified diet based on texturized soy protein was developed for this study. In this model, we studied several bio-markers of zinc deficiency. These include measurement of zinc in plasma, red blood cells, lymphocytes, granulocytes and urine; assay of the following enzymes: deoxythymidine kinase activity in collagen connective tissue harvested following an implantation of sponge under the skin, ecto 5' nucleotidase (5'NT) in lymphocytes (a marker of maturity of lymphocytes) and neutrophil alkaline phosphatase; serum active thymulin; generation of Th1 cytokines Il-2 and IFN-γ; and assay of mRNAs of Th1 cytokines in stimulated cells. Deoxythymidine kinase is required for DNA synthesis in S phase and is essential for cell division. The results showed that the assay of this enzyme is an excellent bio-marker of zinc deficiency in humans. However, this assay is impractical for routine assay.

5'NT, a zinc dependent enzyme is an integral plasma membrane enzyme present in most mammal cells. We assayed 5'

NT activity in the lymphocytes in our experimental subjects. A decrease in the activity of 5'NT was observed in the early depletion phase. Zinc levels in lymphocytes, granulocytes, and platelets decreased significantly only during the late zinc depletion phase. Plasma zinc level did not change even during the late zinc depletion phase. Our studies showed that 5'NT activity is a sensitive and useful bio-marker of human zinc deficiency. A decreased activity of 5'NT in zinc deficient lymphocytes may be indicative of lymphocytes immaturity in human zinc deficiency.

We later established serum thymulin activity, a well characterized thymic hormone, as a bio-marker of human zinc deficiency. Thymulin requires the presence of zinc to express its biological activity. As a result of zinc deficiency the serum active thymulin was decreased and this was corrected by both in vivo and in vitro zinc supplementation suggesting that serum thymulin activity assay was a sensitive bio-marker of zinc deficiency. We also observed that T4+/T8+ ratio was decreased and the generation of IL-2 was decreased and both of these were corrected following zinc supplementation. Inasmuch as thymulin is known to induce intra- and extra thymic T cells differentiation, our studies provided a possible mechanism for the role of zinc on T cell functions. We demonstrated that significant changes in immunological functions due to mild zinc deficiency may be observed in the absence of significant decrease in the plasma zinc concentration, suggesting that the assay of zinc dependent immunologic functions may be better indicators of human zinc deficiency.

Our study showed that the measurement of IL-2 mRNA in peripheral blood MNCs by RT-PCR was a very good indicator of zinc deficiency in humans. We showed that the effect of zinc on the gene expression of IL-2 in the primary cells was because of its role on the activation of NF-κB. Later, we showed that measurement of endogenous zinc excretion may also be a sensitive bio-marker of human zinc deficiency.

Recently, we have shown that the measurement of nail zinc by laser induced background spectroscopy may be an excellent bio-marker of chronic zinc deficiency in humans.

Conclusion: Overall, therapeutic impact of zinc in human health is also overwhelming.

BLACKBERRY JUICE´S PROTECTIVE EFFECT IN RATS UNDER A HYPERCALORIC DIET

Pérez-Grijalva B[1], Mora-Escobedo R[1*], Guzmán-Gerónimo RI[2], Perez-Cruz C[3]

[1]Escuela Nacional de Ciencias Biológicas, Instituto Politécnico Nacional; [2]Instituto de Ciencias Básicas, Universidad Veracruzana; [3]Neuroplasticity and Neurodegeneretion Lab, CINVESTAV, México City, México

Keywords: blackberry juice, microwaves, ultrasound, anthocyanins, metabolic and cognitive deficits

Background: Recent studies have shown that hyperglycemia and hyperinsulinemia conditions can increase the oxidative stress and inflammatory response, resulting in cellular damage and occurrence of chronic degenerative diseases. Blackberries are fruits rich in polyphenols (mainly anthocyanins) with important anti-hyperglycemic, anti-inflammatory, antioxidant and chemopreventive activities. On the other hand it is well known that the conditions of processing and storage have a direct impact on the content of polyphenols in juice, and therefore it is important to apply technologies as microwaves and ultrasound that minimize damages to the polyphenols content.

Objective: Evaluate the protective effects of blackberry juice obtained by applying microwave (60 seconds, 437 W) and ultrasound (10 minutes, 40% amplitude and 20 kHz) in rats fed a hypercaloric diet (HCD).

Methods: Male Wistar rats (100 ± 20 g) were divided into 2 groups: Control group (LabDiet 5001, n=14) and HCD group (sucrose 30%, n=14), and kept on diets for 3 months. At this stage, metabolic parameters were already altered in HCD group, accompanied by cognitive deficits. Thereafter, each group was divided into 2 sub-groups: one received blackberry juice (25 mg/kg/day of anthocyanins, adjusted weekly for weight changes), and the other plain water during 21 days (n=7, each).

Results: HCD causes hyperglycemia, neuroinflammation in hippocampus, increases oxidative stress, and reduces the number of dendritic spines in the CA1 region of the hippocampus, resulting in memory impairments. The blackberry juice supplementation; however, modified these neuroanatomical and metabolic alterations and the behavioural performance in HCD rats.

Conclusion: Blackberry juice can be a potential therapeutic strategy against metabolic and cognitive deficits induced by high-caloric diets.

EFFICACY OF FUROSAP, A NOVEL *TRIGONELLA FOENUM-GRAECUM* SEED EXTRACT, IN ENHANCING TESTOSTERONE LEVEL AND IMPROVING SPERM PROFILE IN MALE VOLUNTEERS

Debasis Bagchi[1,2], Anand Swaroop[1], Manashi Bagchi[1], Pawan Kumar[3] and Harry G. Preuss[4]

[1]Cepham Research Center, Piscataway, NJ, USA, and [2]University of Houston College of Pharmacy, Houston, TX, USA; [3]Chemical Resources, Panchkula, Haryana, India; [4]Georgetown University Medical Center, Washington, DC, USA

Keywords: Furosap, protodioscin, clinical study, testosterone level, mental alertness, mood

Background: Dietary fiber rich fenugreek (*Trigonella foenum-graecum*) seeds have exhibited cardioprotective, hypolipidemic and other health benefits. In our laboratories, we have developed Furosap, an innovative, patent-pending 20% protodioscin-enriched extract from fenugreek seeds, which effectively increased testosterone levels, and significantly improved sperm profile, mental alertness, cardiovascular health, mood, libido and quality of life in male volunteers. Testosterone has also been demonstrated to attenuate lean body mass and stronger bones.

Methods: Institutional Review Board (IRB) and other regulatory approvals were obtained for our study. This one-arm, open-labelled study was conducted in 50 male volunteers (age: 35 to 65 years) over a period of 12 weeks to determine the efficacy of Furosap (500 mg/day/subject). This study examined the testosterone levels, sperm profile, sperm morphology, libido and erectile dysfunction, mood and mental alertness and broad spectrum safety parameters.

Results: Free testosterone levels were improved up to 46% in 90% of the study population. 85.4% of the study population showed improvements in sperm counts. Sperm morphology improved in 14.6% of volunteers. Majority of the subjects enrolled in the study demonstrated improvements in mental alertness and mood. Furthermore, cardiovascular health and libido were significantly improved. Extensive safety parameters were evaluated, which included blood chemistry data. No significant changes were observed in serum lipid function, cholesterol, triglyceride, HDL and LDL levels, hemogram (CBC), hepatotoxicity, cardiotoxicity and nephrotoxicity.

Conclusions: Overall, the results demonstrate that Furosap, enriched in 20% protodioscin, is safe and effective in attenuating testosterone levels, healthy sperm profile, mental alertness, cardiovascular health and overall performance in human subjects.

ENZYMATIC SYNTHESIS OF GLYCOSIDES, THEIR FUNCTIONAL CHARACTERIZATION, AND POTENTIAL USES

Doman Kim [1,2], Thanh Hanh Nguyen [2], Jiyoun Kim [1], Jung-Min Ha [1], Dong-Gu Lee [1], Jin-Beom Si [2]

[1]Department of International Agricultural Technology, Seoul National University, [2]Institutes of Green Bio Science & Technology, Seoul National University, Gangwon-do, 25354, Korea

Keywords: Glycosylation, *Leuconostoc mesenteroides*, glucansucrases, acceptor reaction, oligosaccharides

Background: Glycansucrases are enzymes that synthesize either fructans or glucans using sucrose as substrate. They catalyze the transfer of a sucrose-derived glucose or fructose to other carbohydrates or chemicals containing free OH groups, thereby allowing oligosaccharide synthesis. This reaction is referred to as an acceptor reaction. Glycansucrases also catalyze the transfer of mono-, di-, or higher glucose units to other acceptors via a variety of glycosidic linkages. Transglycosylation catalyzed by enzymes from various bacteria has been used to improve physicochemical properties such as water solubility and oxidative stability of various compounds.

Objective: In order to improve water solubility and stabilities of various less soluble functional compounds, we conducted glycosylation of various compounds, structures were determined, and new functions were characterized.

Methods: To improve accepter reaction yields, the experimental response surface method (RSM) data were fitted via the response surface regression procedure using the following second-order polynomial equation: $Y = \beta_0 + \beta_1 x_1 + \beta_2 x_2 + \beta_3 x_3 + \beta_{11} x_1^2 + \beta_{22} x_2^2 + \beta_{33} x_3^2 + \beta_{12} x_1 x_2 + \beta_{13} x_1 x_3 + \beta_{23} x_2 x_3$. Y is the predicted response and x_1, x_2, x_3 are the independent variables. Analysis of variance was used to estimate the statistical parameters. To purify each glycoside twelve milliliters of the concentrate was applied to a 3 cm × 110 cm Sephadex LH-20 column. Then each fraction was subjected to high performance liquid chromatography. The eluents were concentrated at 65°C with a rotary evaporator. Approximately 5 mg of the purified glycoside was dissolved in 250 µL of D_2O and dispensed into 3 mm NMR tubes. NMR spectra were obtained on a Unity Inova 500 spectrometer operating at 600 MHz for ^1H and 125 MHz for ^{13}C at 25°C. Linkage was evaluated using COSY, HSQC, and HMBC. Browning resistance of each glycoside after UV irradiation in an aqueous system, the antioxidant activity of ascorbic acid, or each glycoside was assessed by DPPH radical scavenging, and tyrosinase inhibition activities were studied.

Results: We synthesized various glycosides of the hydroquinone and flavonoids for the improvement of antioxidant activity. Hydroquinone (HQ) functions as a skin whitening agent, but it has the potential to cause dermatitis. We synthesized a novel HQ fructoside (HF), HQ galactoside and HQ glucoside as potential skin whitening agents by reacting glycansucrases from *Leuconostoc mesenteroides* with HQ as an acceptor and sucrose as a donor. HF synthesis was determined using a response surface methodology and HF showed anti-oxidation activities and inhibition against tyrosinase. The IC_{50} of DPPH scavenging activity was 5.83-mM, showing higher anti-oxidant activity compared to β-arbutin (IC_{50} = 6.04-mM). The K_i value of HF (0.67-mM) against tyrosinase was smaller than that of β-arbutin (K_i = 2.8-mM). Astragalin (kaempferol-3-O-β-D-glucopyranoside, Ast) glucosides were synthesized by the acceptor reaction of a dextransucrase produced by *Leuconostoc mesenteroides* with astragalin and sucrose. Each glucoside was purified and their structures were assigned as kaempferol-3-O-β-D-glucopyranosyl-(1→3)-O-α-D-glucopyranoside (or kaempferol-3-O-β-D-nigeroside, Ast-G1') and kaempferol-3-O-β-D-glucopyranosyl-(1→6)-O-α-D-glucopyranoside (or kaempferol-3-O-β-D-isomaltoside, Ast-G1) for one glucose transferred, and kaempferol-3-O-β-D-isomaltooligosacharide (Ast-IMO or Ast-Gn; n = 2-8). The astragalin glucosides exhibited 8.3-50.6% higher inhibitory effects on matrix metalloproteinase-1 expression, 18.8-20.3% increased antioxidant effects, and 3.8-18.8% increased inhibition activity of melanin synthesis compared to control (without the addition of compound), depending on the number of glucosyl residues linked to astragalin.

Conclusion: Various flavonoids, chemical compounds and carbohydrates glycosides were synthesized by the acceptor reaction of a glycansucrases. Each glycoside was purified and its structure was determined by using nuclear magnetic resonance (NMR). The optimum condition for each glycoside synthesis was determined using a response surface methodology (RSM). Compared to commercial cosmetic functional ingredient, β-arbutin, each glycoside showed varied and/or improved properties depending on the number of glycosyl residues linked to flavonoids. These novel compounds could be used to further expand the industrial applications of various glycosides, particularly in the cosmetics industry.

XYLITOL PRODUCTION FROM WASTE XYLOSE MOTHER LIQUOR CONTAINING MISCELLANEOUS SUGARS AND INHIBITORS: ONE-POT BIOTRANSFORMATION BY *CANDIDA TROPICALIS* AND RECOMBINANT *BACILLUS SUBTILIS*

Hengwei Wang[1], Hairong Cheng[2] and Zixin Deng[2]

[1]Innovation and Application Institute (IAI), Zhejiang Ocean University, Zhoushan 316022, China; [2]State Key Laboratory of Microbial Metabolism, School of Life Sciences and Biotechnology, Shanghai Jiao Tong University, Shanghai 200240, China.

Keywords: Waste xylose mother liquor, One-pot biotransformation, Xylitol, *Candida tropicalis*, *Bacillus subtilis*

Background: Xylitol is one of the functional sugar alcohols. The process of industrial xylitol production is a massive source of organic pollutants, such as waste xylose mother liquor (WXML), a viscous reddish-brown liquid. Currently, WXML is difficult to reuse due to its miscellaneous low-cost sugars, high content of inhibitors and complex composition. WXML, as an organic pollutant of hemicellulosic hydrolysates, accumulates and has become an issue of industrial concern in China. Previous studies have focused only on the catalysis of xylose in the hydrolysates into xylitol using one strain, without considering the removal of other miscellaneous sugars, thus creating an obstacle to subsequent large-scale purification.

Objective: In the present study, we aimed to develop a simple one-pot biotransformation to produce high-purity xylitol from WXML to improve its economic value.

Methods: In the present study, we developed a procedure to produce xylitol from WXML, which combines detoxification, biotransformation and removal of by-product sugars (purification) in one bioreactor using two complementary strains, *Candida tropicalis* X828 and *Bacillus subtilis* Bs12. At the first stage of micro-aerobic biotransformation, the yeast cells were allowed to grow and metabolized glucose and the inhibitors furfural and hydroxymethyl furfural (HMF), and converted xylose into xylitol. At the second stage of aerobic biotransformation, *B. subtilis* Bs12 was activated and depleted the by-product sugars.

Results: The one-pot process was successfully scaled up from shake flasks to 5, 150 L and 30 m3 bioreactors. Approximately 95 g/L of pure xylitol could be obtained from the medium containing 400 g/L of WXML at a yield of 0.75 g/g xylose consumed, and the by-product sugars glucose, l-arabinose and galactose were depleted simultaneously (Figure 1). Finally, xylitol was efficiently crystallized from this bioremoval fermentation.

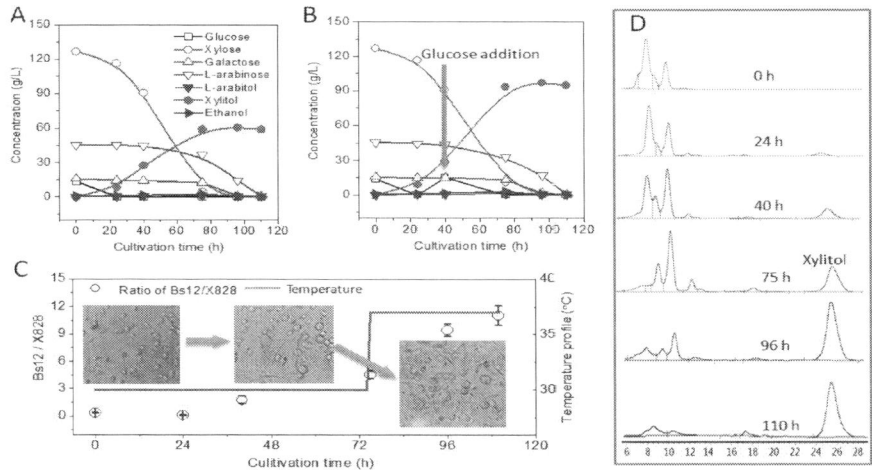

Figure 1. Complementary biotransformation of WXML by *C. tropicalis* X828 and *B. subtilis* Bs12 in shake flasks. (A) and (B), batch biotransformation and glucose fed-batch biotransformation; (C) Ratio of strain Bs12 and X828 cells in glucose fed-batch biotransformation; (D) HPLC profiles of xylitol production.

Conclusions: Our results demonstrate that the one-pot procedure is a viable option for the industrial application of WXML to produce value-added chemicals. The integration of complementary strains in the biotransformation of hemicellulosic hydrolysates is efficient under optimized conditions. Moreover, our study of one-pot biotransformation also provides useful information on the combination of biotechnological processes for the biotransformation of other compounds.

PUERARIN AND ISOflAVONES FROM KUDZU ROOT (PUERARIA LOBATA OHWI) PREVENT ACUTE DRUNKENNESS AND RELIEVE ALCOHOLISM IN MICE

Hongying Lin[1] and Dongrui Zhou[2]

[1]Food Science School, Nanjing Xiaozhuang College, Nanjing, 21000, China; [2]Research Center for Learning Science, Southeast University, Nanjing 210096, China

Keywords: puerarin, kudzu root isoflavones, mice, anti-drunk, drunk time, sober-up time

Background: Puerarin is beginning in the cold-induced febride, all previous dynasties materia medica are recorded, today for crude drugs commonly used, are listed in the "both food and medicine" at the national institutes of health. Puerarin contain a variety of effective components, mainly for the isoflavone compounds: daidzein yuan (daidzein), daidzein (daidzin), 4, 7 - two glucose, daidzein, 3 '- methoxy puerarin, 7 - xylose puerarin, 4', 6 '- diethyl phthalein base a puerarin, etc., but with the highest content of puerarin. Recorded in Chinese pharmacopeia 2010, puerarin flavour GanXin, sexual cold, into the spleen, stomach, lung, a solution of muscle antifebrile, thirst quenching, rash, sun Microsystems antidiarrheal t2dm was bright and poison the function of therapy. Puerarin as traditional Chinese medicine is one of the most representative drug therapies, with ethanol solution wine, for drunkeness, improving cardiovascular circulation, reducing myocardial oxygen consumption, lowering blood sugar, preventing high blood pressure and hardening of the arteries, liver poison resistance, anti-inflammatory, expectorant, antipyretic, improving immunity, antibacterial, antiviral and so on. The many kinds of pharmacological action, can effectively improve liver alcohol dehydrogenase (ADH) and aldehyde dehydrogenase

(ALDH) activity, its function is associated with the biological transformation of enhancing ethanol solution wine, absorption, metabolism, excretion from ethanol three links play a role of therapy, on acute and chronic alcohol poisoning can play a role in therapy. So far, the puerarin therapy towards more acute and chronic alcohol poisoning model under the effect of radix puerariae to protect the liver and other, but for acute therapy anti-drunk research had little effect. In addition, the studies of the effect of puerarin therapy against drunk composition is very few, and the market for acute prevention of drunken hangover, clear effect cure, composition and clear product demand is growing. Based on this situation, this experiment studied the puerarin in mice with acute drunkeness the effect of therapy and prevention effect.

Objective: The present research aimed to evaluate the effects of puerarin and isoflavones from kudzu root (*Pueraria lobata* Ohwi) on preventing acute drunkenness and relieving alcoholism in mice.

Method: First, mice were divided randomly into five groups: control, crude kudzu root extract, kudzu root isoflavone, 60% puerarin, and 99% puerarin. After 12 hours of fasting but with access to water, the mice in each group were orally administered with an equal dose of the corresponding materials in 50% aqueous propylene glycol solution (the solvent alone for the control group). After 30 minutes, the mice from each group were administered by gavage with an identical volume of 56° red star Erguotou liquor. The preventive effect of different contents of puerarin on acute drunkenness was investigated by observing the drunk time and sober-up time. At the same time, the ethanol concentration in blood samples of mice was continuously detected to characterize the degree of intoxication in mice at different time points. Secondly, another batch of mice were divided into four groups, which were administered with kudzu root isoflavone containing approximately 22.13% puerarin at doses of 100, 200, 300 and 400 mg/kg bw after 12 hours of fasting with access to water, respectively. The optimal dose for preventing acute drunkenness and relieving alcoholism was selected based on the drunk time and sober-up time.

Results: With increasing amount of puerarin in the materials administered to mice, the drunk time was increased and sober-up time was shortened. Hence, the effect of puerarin is positively proportional to its content. However, no obvious change was observed when the puerarin content exceeded 300 mg/kg bw.

Conclusion: Puerarin is effective at preventing acute drunkenness and relieving alcoholism. Other isoflavones from kudzu root have similar effect to that of puerarin.

DEHYDRATED MELONS CONTAINING ANTIOXIDANTS FROM GRAPE JUICE

Hulda N. M. Chambi and Flávio L. Schmidt

Department of Food Technology, Faculty of Food Engineering, State University of Campinas, UNICAMP, Campinas, SP 13083-862, Brazil

Keywords: vacuum osmotic dehydration, antioxidant capacity, fruit juice concentrate

Background: Grape juice has a high antioxidant potential, capable of fighting oxidative processes in the body. The juice is marketed mostly in a concentrated form, which has a high content of glucose and fructose. The juice concentrate may be used as an osmotic agent (hypertonic aqueous solution) to dehydrate fruit with a relatively short shelf-life at room temperature, such as melons. The osmotic dehydration process can be carried out at reduced pressures, which must be maintained constant in order to obtain a high dehydration efficiency. This process can be also combined with conventional drying in order to further reduce the water activity of the product

.

Objective: To produce and characterize dehydrated melons with grape juice concentrate (GJC) followed by air-drying.

Methods: Osmotic dehydration was carried out in equipment with natural circulation. Melon (a_w ~0.99, °Brix ~11 and moisture content ~ 88.5%) samples (cubes of 10 mm side) were kept in the grape juice concentrate (60 °Brix) at 40°C under absolute pressure of 600 mbar for 60 minutes using a ratio of fruit to osmotic agents of 1:5, 1:7 and 1:10. The dehydrated melons with the ratio of fruit to osmotic agent of 1:5 were transferred to a forced-air oven kept at 50 °C and 70°C until the melon reached a a_w ~0.7 (25°C). The melon dehydrated with grape juice concertrate followed by an air-drying process along with the melon dehydrated only with grape juice concentrate were evaluated for total phenolics, antioxidant capacity by ABTS, DPPH and ORAC methods, and sensorial acceptance by 60 untrained evaluators. This research was approved by the Research Ethics Committee of State University of Campinas (Brazil) under the number CAAE 41682715.3.0000.5404.

Results: The physical characteristics ($a_w=0.956\pm0.003$, °Brix=31.9±0.5 and moisture content=66.4±1.5 %) of the melon dehydrated using the ratio of 1:5 did not significantly differ from those obtained with other proportions. Dehydration efficiency (water loss/solute gain ~5) was similar for the three processes. These results are interesting since the lower ratio enables the use of less grape juice concentrate in the osmotic dehydration process. The total phenolic content (~4.3 mg of gallic acid equivalent/g sample, d.b) and antioxidant capacity (Table 1) of the dehydrated melon with only grape juice concentrate (dehydrated melon 1) and with grape juice concentrate followed by air-drying process at 50 and 70 °C (dehydrated melon 2 and 3, respectively) showed no significant differences either. This demonstrates that it is possible to combine the two processes to obtain a product with intermediate moisture without decreasing its antioxidant capacity. The samples scored above the acceptable limit (> 5), varying between slightly to moderately, resulted in a purchase intent with average grades between 3 and 4, indicating that there would be a likelihood to purchase the dehydrated melon.

Table 1. Antioxidant capacity

Samples	Antioxidant Capacity (μmol TE/g sample, d.b.)		
	DPPH	ABTS	ORAC
Melon in nature	n.d.	5.5 ± 0.2^d	50.2 ± 4.0^c
GJC	63.2 ± 0.8^a	79.3 ± 2.6^a	320.4 ± 15.9^a
Dehydrated melon 1	15.7 ± 0.5^c	29.0 ± 1.0^b	123.3 ± 3.7^b
Dehydrated melon 2	18.7 ± 0.3^b	27.9 ± 1.7^{bc}	110.4 ± 13.7^b
Dehydrated melon 3	19.4 ± 0.5^b	26.0 ± 0.5^c	94.0 ± 13.4^b

TE – Trolox equivalent; n.d. – non determinated by method. Different superscript letters in the same column indicate significant difference ($p<0.05$).

Conclusion: The study showed that it is possible to use grape juice concentrate to produce dehydrated melons that have antioxidant properties and potential sensory acceptance.

A COMBINATION OF HERBAL EXTRACTS INCREASES LKB1-DEPENDENT ACTIVATION OF AMPK, A RESULT NOT SHARED BY CAMKK2

Jay Whelan[1,2], Dallas Donohoe[1], Yi Zhao[1], E-Chu Huang[1], and Amber MacDonald[1]

[1]Department of Nutrition[1], Agricultural Experiment Station-UTIA[2], University of Tennessee, Knoxville, TN 37996-1920, USA

Keywords: prostate cancer, CWR22, LKB1, CaMKK2, AMPK, herbal extracts

Background: Bioactive natural compounds delivered within a food matrix are involved in molecular multitasking (affecting multiple genomic targets) and deliver their biological punch through biochemical convergence (multiple pathways affecting a common outcome). We demonstrated that these effects occur at physiological concentrations only when the natural products are used in combination. With that, a select blend of herbal extracts (HE) were shown to inhibit growth of tumors in vivo using a preclinical model of castrate-resistant prostate cancer at human equivalent doses. This preparation was comprised of the extracts of 10 herbs: holy basil, turmeric, ginger, green tea, rosemary, hu zhang, barberry, oregano, baikal skullcap, and Chinese goldthread. These effects were mediated, in part, via the activation of AMPK. The role of this pathway has been bolstered as a result of several case studies from MD Anderson Cancer Research Center demonstrating clinical benefit using this select blend of HE, with complementary results from an AMPK activator, metformin.

Objective: To understand the molecular mechanisms responsible for these anti-cancerous effects, we investigated the impact of this blend of HE on upstream and downstream mediators of 5'

adenosine monophosphate-activated protein kinase (AMPK) using a castrate-resistant prostate cancer cell line derived from the CWR22 lineage that produces prostate specific antigen (PSA) and expresses an active androgen receptor, characteristics shared by advanced forms of human prostate cancer.

Methods: CWR22Rv1 cells were treated with and without the HE and protein and/or mRNA levels were measured for downstream biomarkers of AMPK signaling, i.e., mammalian target of rapamycin complex 1 (mTORC1), fatty acid synthase (FASH), acetyl CoA carboxylase (ACC), fatty acid oxidation, and upstream kinases responsible for phosphorylation of AMPK at Ser172 (liver kinase B1, LKB1 and calcium-calmodulin kinase kinase 2, CaMKK2).

Results: When CWR22Rv1 cells were treated with this blend of HE, downstream targets of AMPK were down regulated, i.e., transcription of FASH and SREBP1c (regulator of FASH), with concomitant phosphorylation of ACC (resulting in the negative regulation of fatty acid synthesis) and raptor (regulator of mTORC1). These direct effects of AMPK activation were confirmed by RNAi knockdown, pharmacological inhibition/activation, and overexpression of AMPK. Cellular accumulation of acetyl CoA occurred, along with an increase in fatty acid oxidation. We also observed the concomitant inhibition of the oxidation of glucose. Interrogation of upstream kinases responsible for the activation of AMPK revealed that the HE increases the phosphorylation of PKCzeta (Thr410) and its downstream target LKB1 (Ser428). LKB1's role in the phosphorylation of AMPK was confirmed with RNAi knockdown and pharmacological inhibition. Additional experiments demonstrated that activation of AMPK by the HE was independent of CaMKK2 as confirmed with inhibition studies (BAPTA-AM and STO-609) in the presence and absence of the HE.

These results suggest that combinations of herbal extracts increase AMPK activation via LKB1 and, in turn, decrease lipogenesis at multiple regulatory sites, in addition to downregulating mTOR signaling and the oxidation of glucose, and up regulating fatty acid oxidation.

Conclusion: Bioactives derived from natural products are effective anticancer agents when used at doses in the 20-100 μM range. However, the effective dose is reduced to low nM concentrations when used in combination, underscoring the synergistic action with multiple targets when provided within a more complex matrix. This group of herbal extracts has been shown to inhibit the growth of castrate-resistant prostate cancer cells by activating AMPK signaling. Activation of AMPK by the HE was related to the activation of LKB1, but not CaMKK2. Activation of this pathway was also correlated with an increase in fatty acid oxidation and a reduction in the oxidation of glucose and fatty acid synthesis.

COLONIC DELIVERY OF NUTRIENTS FOR MANAGEMENT OF BLOOD GLUCOSE IN TYPE 2 DIABETES PATIENTS

Jerzy Szewczyk[1], Roger Nolan[1], JoAnn Giannone[1], Stefano Marcuard[2], and Tammy Kindel[3]

[1]BioKier, Inc. Chapel Hill, North Carolina 27514, USA; [2]Carolina Digestive Diseases; Greenville, North Carolina 27834, USA; [3]Department of Surgery, Medical College of Wisconsin, 8701 Watertown Plank Rd, Milwaukee, WI, 53226, USA

Keywords: Diabetes, nutrients, gut hormones, GLP-1, secretagogues, glucose management

Background: It is now widely accepted that malabsorptive surgeries like RYGB, BPD, BPD with duodenal switch and, more recently, the use of the endoluminal sleeve, resolve or improve diabetes. It has been suggested that an increase in gut hormone secretion following surgery or sleeve implantation is the most likely reason for this effect. Expedited delivery of nutrients, such as L-glutamine and butyrate, to the distal small intestine and colon, where most GLP-1 secreting L-cells are expressed, could explain this increase. Validation of this hypothesis would constitute an important step towards developing new therapeutic approaches for treatment of diabetes that take advantage of these physiologic responses.

Objective: To validate the hypothesis that delivery of certain nutrients to the colon causes increased secretion of gut hormones, most importantly GLP-1, we investigated the effects of colonic delivery of nutrients in diabetes. To this end, pre-clinical studies in an animal model of diabetes and clinical studies in type 2 diabetes patients were conducted.

Methods: 10-11 week-old Zucker Diabetic Fatty (ZDF) rats were treated by infusion of sodium butyrate or saline into the colon. Changes in plasma GLP-1 were measured after an oral glucose challenge. Subsequently, 7 week-old ZDF rats (pre-diabetic) were treated chronically with colon-targeted sustained-release butyrate tablets (10mg and 40mg BID) or placebo. Daily basal glucose and weekly basal insulin were measured. Type 2 diabetes patients were treated by infusion of single doses of sodium butyrate, L-glutamine, or placebo into the colon in a double-blinded, cross-over design study. Secretion of GLP-1 and insulin after an oral glucose tolerance test (OGTT) were measured.

Results: Infusion of 4.4mg of sodium butyrate into the colon of ZDF rats restored the GLP-1 secretion after an intra-duodenal glucose challenge. There was no GLP-1 secretion when saline was dose into the colon.

In a chronic study, oral dosing of 40mg of sodium butyrate BID, formulated as colon-targeted sustained-release tablets, completely prevented development of diabetes in ZDF rats; 10mg of butyrate BID significantly slowed progress of the disease. Both doses were effective in improving insulin sensitivity. The placebo group, as well as sham-dosed and untreated control groups, developed diabetes, as routinely observed in this model.

In ten type 2 diabetes patients, being treated with 1-3 anti-diabetes medications (most treated with metformin), infusion of 1g of L-glutamine into the colon caused an increase in GLP-1 (Cmax $p=0.017$ at 30min) and insulin ($p<0.01$ at 90min; $p=0.001$ at 120min; AUC $p<0.005$) secretion after an OGTT. Butyrate increased only insulin secretion at 120min ($p<0.05$). In a pilot study in three metformin-naïve type 2 diabetes patients, both L-glutamine and butyrate were effective in restoring GLP-1 secretion and augmenting insulin secretion, albeit L-glutamine being more effective.

Conclusion: The preclinical studies confirmed the principle, using butyrate as a model compound, that infusion of a nutrient into the colon is able to restore GLP-1 secretion in diabetes. Furthermore, the prevention of elevated glucose levels and an improvement in insulin sensitivity by chronic oral dosing of the gut hormone secretagogue butyrate to the colon of diabetes-prone rats proved the concept that a colon-targeted nutrient could be the basis for an anti-diabetes treatment.

In studies in type 2 diabetes patients to confirm gut hormone secretagogue activity of nutrients, L-glutamine was more effective than butyrate in augmenting secretion of GLP-1 and insulin when infused into the colon. Targeting delivery of L-glutamine to the colon appears to be important because the effects of 1g glutamine delivered to the colon (present study) were greater than the effects of 30g of unformulated glutamine delivered orally (lit. report).

These results suggest that colon-targeted sustained-release delivery of L-glutamine should be very effective in helping patients with type 2 diabetes, who are not able to control their disease with prescription medication, manage their daily glucose. BioKier has developed an oral colon-targeted sustained-release L-glutamine capsule. Because L-glutamine and all components of capsule formulation are GRAS this product could be marketed as a medical food.

PHARMACOKINETIC OF ^{3}H-DEACETYLASPERULOSIDIC ACID IN MICE

Johannes Westendorf[1], Simla Basar-Maurer[1], Thomas Hackl[2], and Edzard Schwedhelm[3]

[1]Institute of Experimental Pharmacology and Toxicology University Medical School, Hamburg-Eppendorf, Martinistrasse 52, D-20461 Hamburg, Germany; [2]University of Hamburg, Institute of Chemistry, Department of NMR-Spectroscopy, Martin-Luther-King Platz 6, D-20146 Hamburg, Germany; [3]Institute of Clinical Pharmacology and Toxicology,University Medical School Hamburg-Eppendorf, Martinistrasse 52, D-20461 Hamburg, Germany

Keywords: Deacetylasperulosidic acid, DAA, tritium label, pharmacokinetic, iridoid, metabolism

Background: Iridoids are a chemical group of secondary plant metabolites with hundreds of different derivatives, which occur in many species of angiosperms, in particular of the superorder of Sympetalae. Most iridoids share a cyclopentanoid monoterpene aglycone attached to a sugar moiety. Some plants use iridoids as precursors for the synthesis of alkaloids but also as a defense against predators. The toxicity of the iridoids depends on its hydrolysis by glycosidases present in the GI-tract or other tissues of animals. The lactone ring of iridoid aglycones can open to form highly reactive dialdehydes, which are able to form adducts with proteins and other functional macromolecules. This can cause toxic effects to the intestinal wall and inner organs of the plant predators. Free carboxylic groups in the C6-position of the six-membered lactone ring, which is the case with DAA, favor the ring opening reaction and enhance the reactivity of the aglycone.

Objective: To understand the lack of toxicity of the plant defense compound deacetylasperulosidic acid (DAA), an iridoid with a highly reactive aglycone, in mammalian species.

Methods: DAA was extracted from *Morinda citrifolia* leaf and purified by preparative HPLC. The identity was verified by MS and NMR spectroscopy. A sample of DAA was radioactively labelled with tritium and applied to mice by gavage. The pharmacokinetic of the radioactivity was investigated in blood, organs, urine and feces. Metabolites were isolated in blood and urine by HPLC and identified by LC-MS. In vitro incubation of DAA with mouse duodenum and liver homogenate and human fecal bacteria was performed and possible metabolites were separated with HPLC.

Results: DAA was rapidly absorbed and excreted mainly via the kidneys with a half-life of 30 minutes. Radioactivity was present in all organs with highest concentrations in kidney and liver. Almost 100% of the radioactivity isolated from urine and organs could be identified as unchanged DAA. Additionally, no metabolism could be observed after in vitro incubation of DAA with mouse small intestine or liver homogenate, indicating that the mammalian glycosidases are not able to hydrolyze the glycosidic bond of DAA; however, a total breakdown of the molecule was observed after incubation of DAA with human intestinal bacteria.

Conclusions: The absorption and excretion of glycosides such as DAA in mammals without hydrolysis is possibly a defense mechanism of animals against the toxicity of these compounds. The total lack of toxicity of DAA in animals and humans suggests that the resistance against the toxicity was acquired early in evolution.

ANTIOXIDANT COFFEE DIETARY FIBER FOR GASTROINTESTINAL HEALTH AND DIABETES

Kenia Vázquez Sánchez[1], Nuria Martinez-Saez[2], Ma. Dolores del Castillo[2], Rocio Campos Vega[1]

[1]Programa en Alimentos del Centro de la Republica (PROPAC), Facultad de Química, Universidad Autónoma de Querétaro, Querétaro, Qro 76010, México. [2]Instituto de Investigación de Ciencias de la Alimentación (CIAL, CSIC-UAM), 28049 Madrid, España.

Keywords: spent coffee grounds, antioxidant dietary fiber, α-glucosidase, gastrointestinal health and diabetes

Background: Spent coffee grounds are a natural sustainable source of antioxidant dietary fiber. The intake of antioxidant dietary fiber has been recommended for health improvement. The transportation of dietary antioxidants through the gastrointestinal tract has been described as an essential function of dietary fiber. Polyphenols linked to dietary fiber may be released in the colon by the action of bacterial microbiota, producing bioactive metabolites and an antioxidant environment, thereby reducing the risk of gastrointestinal diseases associated with oxidative stress and inflammation. The presence of dietary fiber and polyphenols has also been reported to decrease the estimated glycemic index.

Objective: The aim of this study was to evaluate the potential of antioxidant coffee dietary fiber extracted from spent coffee grounds by ohmic treatment as a functional ingredient for gastrointestinal health and diabetes.

Methods: Antioxidant dietary fiber was obtained from spent coffee grounds (ASCGDF, antioxidant spent coffee grounds dietary fiber) by ohmic heating and was incorporated as a food ingredient in biscuit formulations. The microbiological safety of the ingredient was determined previous to its food application. Foods containing 3 and 5 g of coffee fiber were prepared. Control biscuits without addition of dietary fiber were also prepared. A sample of coffee dietary fiber was analyzed in order to estimate its contribution to the health promoting properties of the foods. Coffee antioxidant dietary fiber and biscuits were digested *in vitro* under physiological human gastrointestinal conditions (mouth to colon). The content of bioaccessible free amino groups, fluorescent and total advance glycation end products (AGEs), and antioxidants in the small intestine was determined. The overall antioxidant capacity of the non-digestible fraction (colonic) of the samples was analyzed by direct ABTS (QUENCHER), while the content of bioaccessible antioxidants was analyzed by ABTS under standard conditions. The effect of compounds present in the small intestine on the enzymatic activity of α-glucosidase was measured as indicator of the potential of the coffee antioxidant dietary fiber as a natural source of antidiabetic compounds.

Results: Safety of the coffee antioxidant dietary fiber was confirmed by microbiological analysis. The addition of coffee fiber as a food ingredient increased the overall antioxidant capacity of the foods in a doses depending manner. Most of the antioxidants forming the ingredient and foods remained in the non-digestible fraction (colonic). Lower concentration of AGEs were found in the digests of biscuits containing coffee dietary fiber compared to that corresponding to control food. Inhibitors of alfa-glucosidase were released during digestion of the foods (Table 1).

Table 1. Evaluation of released compounds during the digestion of samples.

Parameters	SCG	ASCGDF	CB	3gB	5gB
Antioxidant capacity (AC)[1]	74.5 ± 3.5^a	54.9 ± 2.5^b	5.4 ± 0.1^c	6.0 ± 0.05^c	6.5 ± 0.03^c
Digestible fraction (small intestine) (AC)[1]	60.1 ± 1.9^a	29.4 ± 0.2^b	23.3 ± 0.6^b	21.9 ± 2.1^b	21.9 ± 1.1^b
Non-digestible fraction (colonic) (AC)[1]	53.4 ± 0.1^a	44.8 ± 1.8^b	31.0 ± 0.5^d	35.0 ± 0.4^c	$32.7 \pm 0.9^{c,d}$
Free amino groups[2]	462.4 ± 18.1^a	410.8 ± 18.1^a	382.1 ± 12.3^a	376.0 ± 1.8^a	371.7 ± 22.9^a
Fluorescent AGEs[3]	$494,362.5 \pm 13,262.5^a$	$1,088,637 \pm 277112.5^b$	$203,125 \pm 5075^c$	$229,937.5 \pm 10687.5^c$	$237,287.5 \pm 29037.5^c$
Total AGEs[4]	459 ± 200.9^b	447 ± 45.3^b	2186 ± 215.4^a	567 ± 74.7^b	510 ± 239.6^b
Enzymatic activity of α-glucosidase (IC_{50})[5]	6.5^a	6.3^a	9.2^a	7.9^a	5.8^a

Means in a row with different letters are significantly different ($p < 0.05$) by Tukey test. Results are expressed as: [1] mg eq CGA / g sample; [2] mM N-α-Lys/g sample; [3] units of fluorescence/ g sample; [4] mU / mL sample; [5] mg / mL sample. **IC$_{50}$**, half maximal α-glucosidase inhibitory activity, **SCG**, spent coffee grounds; **ASCGDF**, antioxidant spent coffee grounds dietary fiber; **CB**, control biscuit; **3gB** and **5gB**, biscuits with 3 and 5 g of ASCDF / serving.

Conclusion: The coffee antioxidant dietary fiber may reach the colon providing some protection against the risk of gastrointestinal diseases associated to oxidative stress. Moreover, during the digestion of the foods containing coffee dietary fiber some compounds may be released in the small intestine able to exert a positive control in the metabolism of sugars making foods friendly for diabetics. *In vivo* studies are needed to confirm the results.

STUDY ON THE IMMUNE FUNCTION OF THE MICE WITH THE *SCHISANDRA CHINENSIS* FERMENTED WINE

Linzheng Lyu and Lanwei Zhang

[1]School of Chemistry and Chemical Engineering, Harbin Institute of Technology, Harbin, 150090, China

Keywords: *Schisandra* fermented wine, fermentation characteristics, immune function

Background: In China, *Schisandra Chinensis* is a resource of traditional medicine food homology, which is usually made into liqueur. In recent years, its fermented wine has become a new development trend. Schizandrin, one active ingredient of *Schisandra Chinensis*, can be enhanced during the fermentation process. But meanwhile, it is confused if the immune function can be enhanced. Therefore it is important to explore the increasing immune function of *Schisandra* fermented wine.

Objective: Through studying the characteristics of fermentation, the experiment showed that there is one good strain to Schisandra fermented wine. Through the fermentation process, the content of Schizandrin will increase. By animal experiments we also wanted to confirm that *Schisandra* fermented wine has good enhancement and protection function on mice immune function. On the whole, this article provides certain theoretical basis for the development and commercialization of *Schisandra* fermented wine.

Methods: *Schisandra* wine is fermented by yeast in 37°C, 2% inoculation quantity, 1:1 inoculation in Schisandra puree. Through the determination of degree of alcohol, the content of flavor substances, effective components, one strain was screened out.

Effective components was determined by HPLC. Then we carried on with the animal experiment. 120 Male ICR mice, body weight was 18 ~ 22 g, feeding temperature was 21±1°C, the humidity was 60±5%, light 12 h/d. Mice were randomly divided into 6 groups after feeding 7 d, with 20 rats in each group respectively as the blank control group, schisandra puree group (200 mg / kg), alcohol control group, low, medium and high Schisandra fermented wine group (100, 200 and 400 mg / kg). Mice were orally administered all doses of solution for 30 days. Determination of index were IgA and IgM levels, immune organ index of spleen and thymus index, determination of the ability of carbon clearance in mice. Data was processed using SPSS statistical software.

Results: For the thymus index, the thymus index of the mice in the high dose group was the highest. For the spleen index, the spleen index of the mice in the high dose group was the highest. Compared to the blank control group, the carbon clearance index increased in each dose group of *Schisandra Chinensis* fermented wine. Compared to the group of *Schisandra* puree, each dose group of carbon clearance index were improved. Clearance ability of mice serum increased with the rise of the dose and high dose group mice had the highest correction carbon clearance index. Compared to the blank control group and alcohol control group, the IgM content of mice was increased in each dose group of *Schisandra Chinensis* fermented wine. Compared to the *Schisandra* puree group, IgM content in each dose group of *Schisandra Chinensis* fermented wine mice were higher and the serum IgM content in middle dose group was the highest. The method of determination of serum IgA levels in mice was ELISA. Compared to the blank control group and alcohol control group, the content of IgA in each dose group increased significantly. Compared to the group of *Schisandra* puree, IgA in each dose group increased and the content of IgA increased by 120.24 μg/ml in middle dose group.

Conclusion: This paper discusses the effect of *Schisandra Chinensis* fermented wine and *Schisandra* fruit puree on immune function in mice from the immune organs, mononuclear macrophage, IgM and IgA content. To sum up, *Schisandra Chinensis* fermented wine can enhance the immune function of mice and its function is better than that of *Schisandra* fruit puree. *Schisandra* fermented wine can enhance the immune function of mice.

COFFEE SILVERSKIN EXTRACT PROTECTS AGAINST BENZO (A) PYRENE INDUCED DNA DAMAGE

Amaia Iriondo-DeHond[1], Ana Haza[2], Alicia Ávalos[2], María Dolores del Castillo[1] and Paloma Morales[2]

[1]Department of Food Analysis and Bioactivity, Institute of Food Science Research (CIAL, CSIC-UAM), 28049 Madrid, Spain; [2] Department of Nutrition, Food Science and Food Technology, Faculty of Veterinary, Universidad Complutense de Madrid, 28040 Madrid, Spain

Keywords: benzo (a) pyrene, chemoprevention, chlorogenic acid, coffee silverskin, DNA bases oxidative damage, genotoxicity

Background: Benzo(a)pyrene also called B(a)P is a chemical carcinogen present in cigarette smoke and in thermally processed foods. B(a)P acts as a genotoxic carcinogen by forming DNA adducts. Several scientific reports have showed the usefulness of plant extracts in the prevention of B(a)P induced cancer in animals by various mechanisms including the prevention of DNA damage and the improvement of the antioxidant status. Coffee silverskin, the only byproduct of coffee roasting, contains phytochemicals possessing antioxidant character such as chlorogenic acid (CGA). The extract (WO/2013/004873) prepared from coffee silverskin (CSE) is enriched in CGA and possesses high antioxidant power. CSE may present chemopreventive potential against B(a)P preventing DNA damage.

Objective: The aim of the present study was to investigate the chemopreventive potential of CSE against B(a)P induced DNA damage in HepG2 cells and to find out the contribution of CGA in CSE as a chemopreventive agent.

Methods: Prior to the evaluation of DNA damage, cytotoxicity of the studied compounds was analyzed using the MTT method. DNA damage (strand breaks and oxidized purines/pyrimidines) was evaluated by the alkaline single-cell gel electrophoresis or comet assay. HepG2 cells were pre-treated with CSE or CGA (1, 10 and 100 µg/ml) for 24 h followed by the addition of 100 µM B(a)P in presence of the chemopreventive agents for another 24 h. Detection of oxidized purines and pyrimidines was carried out using Formamidopyrimidine DNA glycosylase or Endonuclease III enzymes, respectively. Data was expressed as % Tail DNA.

Results: CSE and CGA were not cytotoxic at the tested concentrations (1, 10 and 100 µg/ml). Treatment with 100 µM B(a)P significantly increased ($p < 0.05$) the levels of DNA strand breaks and oxidized purine and pyrimidine bases. CSE significantly inhibited ($p < 0.05$) genotoxicity induced by B(a)P. CGA alone at the concentration present in CSE was effective against B(a)P. CSE chemopreventive effect may be associated to its antioxidant capacity. CGA seems to be a contributor to the chemopreventive effect of CSE against B(a)P induced DNA damage in HepG2 cells.

Conclusion: CSE presents potential as a natural and sustainable chemopreventive agent against the chemical carcinogen B(a)P being a promising candidate as functional food ingredient for cancer. Chemoprevention of cancer by dietary phytochemicals is a promising approach. Further investigation is needed to confirm these preliminary results.

COFFEE SILVERSKIN EXTRACT FOR DIABETES

María Dolores del Castillo[1], Beatriz Fernández-Gomez[1], María Ángeles Martín[2] and María Dolores Mesa[3]

[1]Department of Food Analysis and Bioactivity, Institute of Food Science Research (CIAL, CSIC-UAM), 28049 Madrid, Spain; [2]Department of Nutrition and Metabolism, Institute of Food Science, Technology and Nutrition (ICTAN-CSIC), 28040 Madrid, Spain; [3]Institute of Nutrition and Food Technology "José Mataix", University of Granada, 18100 Granada, Spain

Keywords: Antioxidant capacity, caffeine, chlorogenic acid, coffee silverskin, diabetes, intestinal alpha glucosidase, pancreas oxidative stress

Background: Coffee silverskin is a thin tegument of the outer layer of the two beans forming the green coffee seed that is obtained as a by-product of the roasting product. Our research group patented an aqueous extract of coffee silverskin (CSE) (P2011311128) possessing powerful antioxidant capacity. Oxidative stress and inflammation are intimately linked with the pathogenesis of type 2 diabetes (T2D). An increase in oxidative stress-derived inflammation is a major mechanism in the pathogenesis of diabetes and related diseases such as diabetic nephropathy.

Objective: To get insights in the effects of an aqueous coffee silversin extract in the pathogenesis of diabetes, using diabetic rats.

Methods: *In vivo* antidiabetic effect of CSE, CGA and caffeine was evaluated using an experimental model of streptozotocin-nicotinamide (STZ-NA) induced T2D rats. Thirty-two rats were daily pre-treated with the CSE, CGA or caffeine during 34 days.

At day 35, diabetes was induced by intraperitoneal injection of STZ-NA and blood samples were collected in the fasting state at day 42. After blood centrifugation, plasma was separated and frozen at -80 °C. The pancreas were removed promptly, weighted, divided into three parts and then stored at −80 °C until required. Plasma glucose was measured using a colorimetric kit. As biomarkers of oxidative stress the activity of glutathione peroxidase and glutathione reductase; as well as, the levels of reduced glutathione and pancreatic protein oxidation were measured in homogenates of pancreas. The effect of CSE in the *in vitro* activity of intestinal alpha-glucosidase was also analyzed. Alpha-glucosidase inhibitors appear to be a therapeutic option in the treatment of T2D.

Results: Novel findings were obtained during the development of this investigation. The supplementation of rats with pure CGA and caffeine tended to reduce ($p < 0.1$) STZ-NA-induced oxidation of pancreas proteins. Pre-treatment of animals with CSE and CGA significantly reduced ($p < 0.05$) STZ-induced pancreas GSH depletion. Results confirm the bioavailability of caffeine and CGA in CSE and support their biological implications in diabetes. CSE caused a significant inhibition of the activity of alpha-glucosidase enzyme *in vitro*. More data regarding the antidiabetic effect of CSE are summarized in the patent with number P201431848.

Conclusion: CSE exerts a chemo-protective effect of CSE in pancreatic tissue, and this effect may be associated with its antioxidant capacity. Daily administration of CSE, CGA or caffeine 35 d previous to the induction of diabetes significantly reduced ($p < 0.05$) pancreatic oxidative stress and protein damage. CSE antidiabetic effect can be also associated to its capacity to inhibit intestinal alpha-glucosidase.

TRANSCRIPTION FACTOR EB IS A CRUCIAL TRANSDUCER OF THE BIOMEDICAL ACTION OF PTEROSTILBENE

Martina La Spina[1], Michele Azzolini[2], Andrea Mattarei[3], Giulietta Di Benedetto[2], Cristina Paradisi[3], Mario Zoratti[1,2], Lucia Biasutto[1,2]

[1]Department of Biomedical Sciences of the University of Padua, Padua, 35121, Italy; [2]Institute of Neuroscience of CNR, Padova, Italy; [3]Department of Chemical Sciences, University of Padova, Padua, 35121 Italy

Keywords: Polyphenols, Pterostilbene, Autophagy, cAMP-AMPK/CREB pathway

Background: Polyphenols are a large and diversified class of natural compounds produced by plants in response to stressing conditions. In our laboratory, we focus our attention on stilbenoids and in particular on Pterostilbene (Pt), a di-methylated analogue of much-studied Resveratrol (Rv). Many studies, most of them performed *in vitro,* suggest that Pt has beneficial properties similar to those of Rv. Importantly, Pt is more bioavailable than Rv. In fact, in rats Pt can reach micromolar concentrations in many organs after a single oral administration. Although the striking effects of these two compounds are widely recognized, much remains to be learned about their molecular mechanisms of action. One is thought to be the induction of autophagy. The master regulator of autophagy is Transcription Factor EB (TFEB). Its subcellular localization and activation depend on phosphorylation events. TFEB is normally retained in the cytosol because of an inhibitory phosphorylation by mTORC1 but, under conditions of nutrients deprivation or lysosomal stress, it is dephosphorylated and it can translocate to the nucleus where it regulates the expression of its target genes. The induction of autophagy by polyphenols is well supported. In particular, a pro-autophagic role is already ascribed to Rv.

Objective: To evaluate whether Pt and its main metabolites (DiHydroPt and Pt-4-Sulfate), the main species present in the body after ingestion, may modulate TFEB activity and thus autophagy. In case of a positive answer to the 1st point, how these molecules stimulate TFEB activity.

Methods: To follow TFEB localization, confocal microscopy was carried out on HeLa cells overexpressing TFEB-GFP (kindly provided by Prof. Ballabio of TIGEM-Naples), treated or not with stilbenoids. RT-qPCR analyses were performed to check the transcription levels of some TFEB target genes. Autophagy induction and the activation of some kinases that may regulate the transcription factor were evaluated by Western blotting. Variations of cellular cAMP levels were also measured by using a FRET-based sensor.

Results: TFEB is a key mediator of Pt induced-autophagy: Pt, in our system, triggered TFEB nuclear translocation already at low, physiologically meaningful concentrations but to a lesser extent if compared to starvation. Accordingly, Pt decreased the phosphorylation levels of S6, a mTORC1 target. Moreover, while Pt-4-Sulfate, a phase II metabolite, was almost ineffective, DiHydroPt, formed by gut microbiota, showed an activity similar to that of the parent compound. Treatment with Pt or DiHydroPt also revealed an upregulation of some selected TFEB target genes, as reported by RT-qPCR. Western Blotting analysis supports the activation of autophagy in cultured HeLa cells, showing an increase in the lipidation of LC3B.

Upstream signaling: the pleiotropic activity of polyphenols is thought to be the consequence of interactions with multiple proteins. Many studies identify AMPK as target of Rv. Rv is reported to indirectly activates AMPK through an increase in cAMP concentration due to the inhibition of some phosphodiesterases (PDE). Thus, we verified whether Pt could modulate cAMP and its downstream signaling as well. FRET based-measurements revealed that Pt promotes an increase in the concentration of this cyclic nucleotide in HeLa cells. Considering the well-recognized antagonistic relationship between AMPK and mTORC1, we next wondered if TFEB translocation may be due to the increase in the concentration of this second messenger and could involve AMPK. The results indicated that Pt-induced TFEB migration is only partly downstream cAMP/AMPK signaling.

Finally, the involvement of cAMP response element binding protein (CREB) was also considered. As expected, Pt induced a rapid and transient increase in the phosphorylation levels of this transcription factor.

Conclusions: As hypothesized, given that polyphenols are able to induce autophagy and considering the key role attributed to TFEB as a master regulator of autophagy, Pt induced migration of TFEB-GFP in HeLa cells overexpressing the chimera. The relocation of the transcription factor was accompanied by an increase of cAMP levels. The involvement of AMPK was tested but our results suggest that this pathway doesn't fully account for the phenomenon. Thus, the induction of autophagy by Pt seems to have more than one effector. Seok et al., in 2014 reported a crucial role also for CREB in the regulation of lipophagy and in the expression of autophagic genes. According to these findings, we observed an increase in the activation of this transcription factor after Pt treatments.

LUTEIN AND ZEAXANTHIN ISOMERS PROTECT PHOTORECEPTORS AGAINST BLUE LIGHT-INDUCED DEGENERATION

Minzhong Yu[1,2], Craig Beight[1]

[1]Department of Ophthalmic Research, Cole Eye Institute, Cleveland Clinic Foundation, Cleveland OH, USA; [2]Department of Ophthalmology, Cleveland Clinic Lerner College of Medicine of Case Western Reserve University, Cleveland OH, USA

Key words: Lutemax 2020, Lutein, Zeaxanthin, Mesozeaxanthin, Oxidative stress, photoreceptor degeneration, Blue light damage; electroretinogram

Background: Oxidative stress is a major factor underlying photoreceptor degeneration. Lutein and zeaxanthin isomers (L/Zi), consisting of lutein, zeaxanthin and mesozeaxanthin carotenoids and found widely in many foods, protect against cell damage by ameliorating oxidative stress in retina.

Objective: In this study, we examined the effect of L/Zi supplementation in a mouse model of light-induced photoreceptor degeneration.

Methods: L/Zi (Lutemax2020, 10 mg/kg) dissolved in sunflower oil (1 mg/ml) or equal volume of sunflower oil as vehicle was administered by daily oral gavage to 2-month old BALBc/J mice in treatment group (n=7) and vehicle group (n=7), respectively for a 5 day period. On Day 2, animals were exposed for 1 hour to blue light (5,000 lux) obtained by filtering white fluorescent light by a filter which transmitted light between 380 and 570 nm (Midnight Blue 5940, Solar Graphics, Clearwater, Florida). Pupils were not dilated and mice were able to move freely during light exposure.

Electroretinograms (ERGs) were recorded prior to light exposure (baseline) and then and then again on Day 8, 1 week after light exposure, after which mice were sacrificed for anatomical analysis.

Results: At baseline, ERG amplitudes were comparable in Li/Zi and vehicle control mice. After light exposure, ERGs were markedly reduced in the vehicle control mice, consistent with prior studies. In comparison, ERGs obtained at baseline and after light exposure were comparable in Li/Zi mice.

Conclusions: Pre-treatment with L/Zi can protect photoreceptors against degeneration induced by high intensity blue light. Future studies will examine the potential for L/Zi in inherited forms of photoreceptor degeneration involving oxidative stress.

Support: Omni Active Health Technologies Ltd., India Research Grant, Research to Prevent Blindness, Foundation Fighting Blindness

THE PROFILE OF POLYPHENOLS AND ANTIOXIDANT CAPACITY OF SELECTED MEDICINAL PLANTS OF BANGLADESH

Nazma Shaheen[1], Avonti Basak Tukun[1], Saiful Islam[1], Nafis Md. Irfan[1], Ishrat Nourin Khan[1] and Thingnganing Longvah[2]

[1]Institute of Nutrition and Food Science, University of Dhaka, Dhaka-1000, Bangladesh; [2]National Institute of Nutrition, Hyderabad, Hyderabad-500 007, India

Keywords: Polyphenol, antioxidant capacity, medicinal plant, DPPH, IC_{50}

Background: Indigenous foods contain a wide variety of phytochemicals including thousands of bioactive compounds, pigments and natural antioxidants. Apart from the consumption as part of the normal diet these indigenous foods go beyond basic nutrition and have scientifically demonstrated specific targeted actions to provide enhancement of the state of well-being and health to improve the quality of life and/or reduce the risk of heart disease, hypertension, diabetes and some form of cancer. But, the indigenous foods of Bangladesh has rarely been documented or explored for their functional components and effects. Over the last decade, the most interesting bioactive compounds with health beneficial effect have been polyphenols.

Objective: The objective of the present study was to screen total phenol content (TPC) and to assess antioxidant capacity (AC) and polyphenol profile of 15 indigenous foods of Bangladesh.

Methods: Collection of fresh samples of 15 food items followed by sample preparation that involved separation of the edible portion, weighing, washing (with running tap water followed by distilled water) and air-drying. Each sample was then freeze-dried at -180°C, weighed, ground and stored in air tight package at -

20°C until they underwent further analysis. Freeze-dried samples were extracted by solid phase extraction method. The Total Phenol Content (TPC) of the selected food items' methanol extracts was determined colorimetrically according to the Folin-Ciocalteau method. Estimation of Antioxidant Activity (AA) in both methanol and water extracts of all the samples was performed by employing 2, 2-diphenyl-1-1-picrylhydrazyl radical scavenging assay (DPPH-RSA) and $IC_{50.}$ Methanol extracts were centrifuged and filtered for simultaneous determination of individual polyphenols. Individual polyphenol standards were used to characterize and quantitate individual polyphenolic compounds by HPLC.

Results: TPC ranged from 276.85 (*Moringa oleifera*) to 15.45 (*Zanthoxylum rhetsa*) mg per 100g. The % DPPH inhibition in methanol and water extract were high in *Zanthoxylum rhetsa* (92.86) and *Moringa oleifera* (91.87) respectively and they also showed the lowest IC_{50} in corresponding solvent system. The lowest % DPPH inhibition was found in *Spilanthes calva* (24.49) and *Centella asiatica* (4.88) in methanol and water extract respectively. Ten individual polyphenols were screened (Chlorogenic acid, coumaric acid, caffeic acid, apigenin-7-o-neohesperidoside, apigenin, querectin-3-beta D-gluoside, querectin-3-o-glucopyranoside, kaemperfrol, isoramanetin, lutelion). *Amaranthus viridis*, *Spilanthes calva*, *Oxalis corniculata*, *Piper retrofractum*, *Moringa oleifera* contained the highest amount of chlorogenic acid, coumaric acid, caffeic acid, apigenin-7-o-neohesperidoside, apigenin respectively. *Senna tora* contained the highest amount of querectin-3-beta D-gluoside, kaemperfrol and isoramanetin respectively whereas querectin-3-o-glucopyranoside and lutelion were highest in *Alternanthera sessilis*.

Conclusion: Moringa oleifera, with lowest IC50 and highest %DPPH inhibition and TPC, was the most potent antioxidant sample among analyzed samples.

EVALUATION OF FUNCTIONAL POTENTIALITY OF SELECTED COMMONLY CONSUMED FOODS OF BANGLADESH

Nazma Shaheen, Avonti Basak Tukun, Saiful Islam, Nafis Md. Irfan, Ishrat Nourin Khan and Towhid Hasan

Institute of Nutrition and Food Science, University of Dhaka, Dhaka-1000, Bangladesh

Keywords: Total phenol content, Antioxidant capacity, Anti-inflammatory activity, Bangladeshi foods

Background: Everyday foods contain a wide variety of phytochemicals including thousands of bioactive compounds, pigments and natural antioxidants. Apart from the consumption as part of the normal diet these indigenous foods go beyond basic nutrition and have scientifically demonstrated specific targeted actions to provide enhancement of the state of well-being and health to improve the quality of life and/or reduce the risk of heart disease, hypertension, diabetes and some form of cancer. But, the indigenous foods of Bangladesh has rarely been documented or explored for their functional components and effects. Over the last decade, the most interesting bioactive compounds with health beneficial effect have been polyphenols.

Objective: The objective of the present study was to screen 73 commonly consumed foods of Bangladesh for total phenol content (TPC) and antioxidant capacity (AC) and determine their anti-inflammatory effects.

Methods: Collection of fresh samples of 73 food items followed by sample preparation that involved separation of the edible portion, weighing, washing (with running tap water followed by distilled water) and air-drying. Each sample was then freeze-dried at -180°C, weighed, ground and stored in an airtight package at -20°C until they underwent further analysis. Freeze-dried samples were sequentially extracted by hexane: dichloromethane (1:1) and acetone:water:acetic acid (AWA) (70:29.5:0.5). The Total Phenol Content (TPC) of the selected food items' AWA extracts was determined colorimetrically according to the modified Folin-Ciocalteau method. Estimation of Antioxidant Activity (AA) in AWA extracts of all the samples was performed by employing 2, 2-diphenyl-1-1-picrylhydrazyl radical scavenging assay (DPPH-RSA) (figure 1). In vitro inflammatory activity was assessed by LPS-induced production on J774A.1 cells of TNF-α an inflammatory cytokine produced in the early phase of inflammation in the DMSO extracts of freeze-dried samples of 41 food items; of which fourteen food items showed to possess anti-inflammatory potential. Dose-response study of these fourteen food items was carried out to further confirm the in vitro inhibition of TNF-α. Finally, in vivo anti-inflammatory potential was identified by carrageenan induced paw edema in rats.

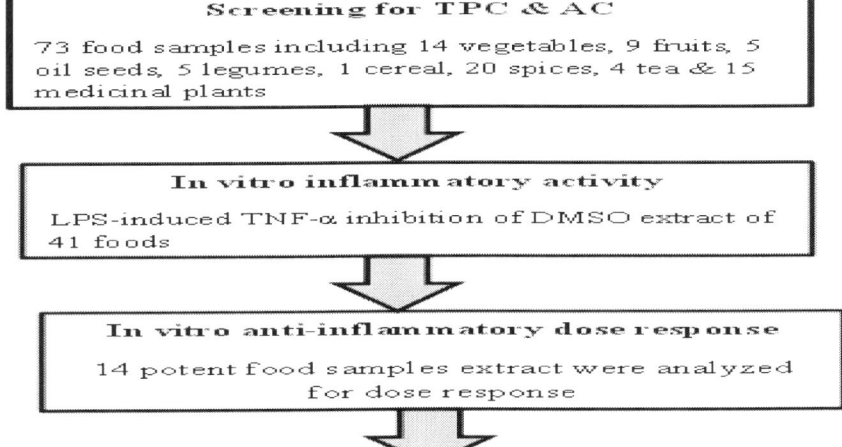

Results: TPC varied in the range of 0.50 (bottle gourd) - 13.91 (egg plant) mg GAE (Gallic acid equivalent)/ g in vegetables, 0.21 (water melon) – 18.97 (wood apple) mg GAE / g in fruits, 1056.74 (tea mirzapur) - 2348.60 (green tea) mg GAE / g in tea samples, 15.92 (sesame brown) - 28.80 (mustard brown) mg GAE / g in oil seeds, 5.93- (lentil)- 13.68 (black gram) mg GAE/g of fresh weight (fw) in legumes and cereal. In spices, TPC varied in the range of 0.39 (garlic) - 49.89 (cloves) mg GAE/ g of dry weight (dw).

Antioxidant activity in terms of DPPH varied in the range 0.75 (cabbage) - 71.86 (tomato) µmole TE (Trolox equivalent)/ g in vegetables, 0.21 (water melon) - 185.78 (Amla) µmole TE/g in fruits, 1269.91 (tea mirzapur) - 2432.76 (green tea) µmole TE/g in tea samples, 8.36 (sesame black)- 356.72 (linseed) in oil seeds, 8.21 (khesari dal) - 617.5 (Cheena) µmole TE/g of fresh weight in legumes and cereal. In spices sample AA varied from 179.21 µmol TE/g of dry weight in Cloves to 0.78 µmol TE/g of dry weight in Garlic.

Two teas, spices and oil seed, all legumes, one vegetable, fruit and cereal samples inhibited TNF-α production at the concentration of 40µg/mL. Among them, activities of linseed (32.3%), cheena (48.85%), kheshari (48.59%), radhuni (49.91%), cabbage (54.21%), black tea (53.4%) and sesame-black variety (57.5%) were potent. Dose response study the inhibition of TNF-α production (40, 10, 3 & 1µg/mL) showed that two spices, green tea, tea organic, sesame (black), mustard (yellow), green gram and lentil seems to have dose-response.

Conclusions: The present study is a useful database for TPC and antioxidant activity in commonly consumed foods of Bangladesh. Several polyphenol rich foods showed both in vitro and in vivo anti-inflammatory activity and confirmed dose-response relationship. Findings of the present study is a significant addition in the food functionality of Bangladeshi foods.

TOPICAL APPLIED NUTRACEUTICAL ANTIOXIDANT FORMULATION REDUCES OCULAR OXIDATIVE STRESS

Peter F. Kador[1,2], Changmei Guo[1], Hiroyoshi Kawada[1], James Randazzo[1] and Karen Blessing[1,2]

[1]Department of Pharmaceutical Sciences, College of Pharmacy, University of Nebraska Medical Center, Omaha, Nebraska, USA
[2]Therapeutic Vision Inc., Omaha, Nebraska, USA

Keywords: oxidative stress, nutraceutical antioxidants, age-related ocular diseases

Background and Objective: Evaluation of oral nutraceutical antioxidants for oxidation induced age-related cataract and other ocular diseases have shown disappointing clinical results. Based on the hypothesis that nutraceuticals do not adequately reach the lens by oral administration, we have developed a unique topical antioxidant formulation whose active ingredients have the reported ability to reduce oxidative stress through free radical scavenging and chelating activity. This formulation mimics the *in vivo* activity of multifunctional antioxidants, compounds being developed in our laboratory that independently scavenge free radicals selectively bind redox metals.

Methods: Oxidative stress was induced in the eyes of rats by 15 min exposure to 1600 $\mu W/cm^2$ of UV light, diabetes by tail vein injection of streptozotocin, and exposure of dark adapted rats to 1000 lx of light. Retinal degeneration was induced in dark-adapted rats by light exposure. Dry eye was induced in rats by subcutaneous scopolamine injections. Glutathione (GSH) levels were spectrophotometrically measured while retinal oxidative stress markers were measured by ELISA and western blot. The topical nutraceutical was administered b.i.d. and compared in select experiments to topical and oral multifunctional antioxidant

JHX-4, oral and topical aldose reductase inhibitors, a veterinary ocular antioxidant formulation and topical hyaluronic acid.

Results: In rats exposed to UV light, the nutraceutical formulation was able to significantly protect lenses against decreased GSH levels induced by exposure to UV light. Similarly, this formulation delayed the progression of cataracts induced by diabetes. In light damaged rats, the topical nutraceutical partially protected the neural retina and photoreceptors against oxidative stress compared to the multifunctional antioxidant. The topical nutraceutical also maintained tear flow in the scopolamine treated rats.

Conclusion: While less potent than the small molecule multifunctional antioxidants that will require FDA approval, the topical nutraceutical formulation beneficially reduces ocular oxidative stress in rats. These studies suggest that this topical antioxidant may fill the unmet therapeutic need of providing a topical antioxidant formulation that delays the progression of cataracts and reduces the risk of AMD.

Supported by a grant from CLC Medica and Therapeutic Vision, Inc.

ANTIBACTERIAL ACTIVITY OF *ILEX PARAGUARIENSIS* (*YERBA MATE*) AGAINST GRAM POSITIVE AND GRAM NEGATIVE BACTERIA

Tania Noureddine[1], Ziad El Husseini[1], Ali Nehma [1], Ziad Daoud[1], Roula M. Abdel-Massih[2]

[1]Laboratory of Microbiology, Faculty of Medicine and Medical Sciences, University of Balamand, Lebanon; [2]Department of Biology, University of Balamand, Lebanon.

Keywords: Antibacterial Activity, Yerba Mate, MIC, MBC

Background: Leaves of the plant *Ilex paraguariensis* are popularly used in South America, and some Middle Eastern countries (such as Lebanon, Syria, etc.) in the preparation of tea infusions (Yerba Mate). Previous literature studies of *Ilex paraguariensis* have displayed a wide range of health benefits as antimutagenic, antiglycation, and antioxidant effects. They were also found to have hepatoprotective, hypocholesteremic and vasodilation effects. Several studies have reported improvement in glycemic and lipidic profile of type 2 diabetes and weight reduction in mice studies after Mate intake. In recent publications, habitual consumption of Yerba Mate has shown neuroprotective, anticonvulsant and anti-depressant effects (1, 2).

Objective: The antibacterial activity of aqueous extract of *Ilex paraguariensis* leaves was assayed on different strains of Gram positive and Gram negative bacteria.

Methods: In the present work, the antibacterial activity of dialyzed aqueous extract of commercial leaves was studied against standard strains of *Staphylococcus aureus* ATCC29213, *Pseudomonas aeruginosa* ATCC 25873, *Acinetobacter baumannii* ATCC 17978 *and Escherichia coli* ATCC 35218. The antibacterial activities of these extracts were also tested against 25 clinical isolates of *Klebsiella pneumonia, Enterococcus faecalis, Enterobacter aerogenes, Enterobacter agglomerans and Serratia marcesens.*

For the extraction, dried leaves of commercial brand of Yerba Mate (Amanda; Argentina; Stems and Leaves 100%; Ilex Paraguariensis) were finely ground to small particles using a food blender. Sterile deionized water was added to the ground leaves and stems at a ratio of 3.6 ml to 1 g of ground Yerba Mate and boiled at 70°C for 2 hours with occasional stirring. The extract was subsequently filtered and then centrifuged at 5000 g for 30 minutes at 4°C. The supernatant was dialyzed against deionized water at 4°C for 48 hours, concentrated at 70°C, and then dried using SpeedVaccum Concentrator. The obtained extract was weighed, dissolved in deionized water at a concentration of 120mg/ml, and stored at 4°C.

For the determination of the Minimum Inhibitory Concentration (MIC) and the Minimum Bactericidal Concentration (MBC), 50µl of the extract solution (120mg/ml) were added to a 150µl of Mueller Hinton Broth. It was then serially diluted according to the broth microdilution method to determine the minimal inhibitory concentration (MIC). A bacterial suspension of 10^6CFU/ml was used to inoculate the wells. After 24 hours of incubation, and after determining the MICs, the tubes with no growth were sub-cultured to determine the MBC.

Results: Antibacterial activity of the Yerba Mate aqueous extract was observed against all tested strains; however, it varied between Gram positive and Gram negative organisms, showing a greater activity against *S. aureus* ATCC29213 and *Enterococcus faecalis* with MIC of 0.468 mg/ml and 0.468 mg/ml and MBC of 0.468 mg/ml and 1.875 mg/ml, respectively. In addition, the extract displayed a high activity against *Acinetobacter baumannii* ATCC 17978 with MIC and MBC 0.468 mg/ml.

The antibacterial activity of the extract did not show any correlation with the profile of resistance of the tested bacteria, *E. coli* ATCC35218 and ESBL producing *E. coli* both had the same MIC (1.875 mg/ml) and MBC (3.750 mg/ml). The MIC for Methicillin Sensitive *S. aureus* and Methicillin Resistant *S. aureus* was also the same (1.875 mg/ml). AmpC producing *E. coli* and OXA-48 producing *E. coli* both exhibited the same MIC and MBC (3.750 mg/ml). In general, the MIC and MBC values ranged between 0.468 mg/ml and 15 mg/ml.

Conclusion: The conclusions from this study suggest that the aqueous extract of *Ilex paraguariensis* exhibits strong antibacterial activity against both Gram positive and Gram negative bacteria. A more in-depth analysis to identify the active molecule responsible for this activity as well as testing a wider range of bacterial isolates is important for a better understanding of the potential role of Yerba Mate in developing new antibacterial agents.

References

1. Bracesco N, Sanchez AG, Contreras V, Menini T, Gugliucci A. Recent advances on *Ilex paraguariensis* research: minireview. J. Ethnopharmacol. 2011, 136 (3):378-84.

2. Rempe CS, Burris KP, Woo HL, Goodrich B, Gosnell DK, Tschaplinski TJ, et al. (2015) Computational Ranking of Yerba Mate Small Molecules Based on Their Predicted Contribution to Antibacterial Activity against Methicillin-Resistant *Staphylococcus aureus*. PLoS ONE 10(5): e0123925. doi:10.1371/journal.pone.0123925

BETA-CRYPTOXANTHIN (BCX) IMPROVES LUNG FUNCTION AND REDUCES STRESS INDUCED INFLAMMATION: *IN VIVO* MODEL

Vijaya Juturu[1,] Kazim Sahin[2], Ragip Pala[2], Mehmet Tuzcu[2], Nurhan Sahin[2] and Oguzhan Ozdemir[2]

[1]Scientific and Clinical Affairs, OmniActive Health Technologies Inc., Morristown, NJ, United States [2]Nutrition and Veterinary, Firat University, Elazig, Turkey

Keywords: Beta-cryptoxanthin, Exercise, Lung function, Oxidative stress, Antioxidant capacity

Background: Beta-cryptoxanthin (BCX) may protect against environmental allergies by reducing oxidative damage and reduces stress induced inflammation. We recently demonstrated that BCX up-regulated E-cadherin (ECAD) in primary bronchial epithelial cells. Strenuous physical exercise is associated with a 10- to 20-fold increase in whole body oxygen consumption and oxidative stress. The lungs are a major target for various inflammatory, oxidative, carcinogenic or infectious stressors, which result in a range of lung diseases.

Objective: To investigate beta-cryptoxanthin (BCX) supplementation on exercise (EX) performance, exhaustion time, and changes in serum, muscle and lung proteins in rats after exhaustive exercise.

Methods: Eight week old male Wistar rats were treated with four treatment groups (i) control [no Ex, Group I (CTL)] (ii) CTL + BCX [no Ex, 2.5 mg BCX [BCXcel], Group II] (iii) CTL + Ex [Group III] and (iv) CTL + Ex+ BCX [Ex, 2.5 mg BCX [BCXcel], Group IV] administered daily for 8 wks. The Ex protocols were performed on a motor-driven rodent treadmill (TMR). The animals in the chronic Ex groups habituated by treadmill Ex over a 5-d period such as: 1st day 10 m/min, 10 min, 2nd day 20 m/min; 10 min, 3rd day 25 m/min, 10 min, 4th day 25 m/min, 20 min and 5th day 25 m/min, 30 min. Animals were exercised at 25 m/min, 45 min/d, 5 d/ week for 8 wks. Blood analysis for triglycerides (TG) and cholesterol (CHOL), muscle analysis for lactate, muscle and lung antioxidant capacity (SOD, GPx), muscle and lung oxidative stress (OS, MDA) was analyzed. Gene protein levels such as NFκB, Nrf2 and HO1 were analyzed in each group of rats by real time RT-PCR and Western blotting.

Results: Group IV significantly increased running performance and exhaustion time. In Group IV a significant decrease in TG and CHOL were observed compared with other treatments. A significant decrease in lactate, muscle oxidative stress and increase in muscle antioxidant activity observed in Group IV. Protein levels of nuclear factor (erythroid-derived 2)-like 2 (Nrf2), and heme oxygenase-*1* (HO1) increased and a decrease in nuclear factor (NFκB) was observed in Group IV. There were no significant differences in any of the end points in Group I and II. No significant changes in liver and kidney functions were observed in any of the treated groups.

Conclusion: The present data suggest that BCX enhances exhaustion time and decreases OS. These results suggest BCX with Ex may enhance the exhaustion time by regulating HO1 and Nrf2 exerts anti-oxidant, anti-inflammatory and anti-apoptotic properties via its reaction products.

ANSERINE DIPEPTIDE FROM FISH EXTRACTS AMELIORATE THE URIC ACID LEVELS IN FRUCTOSE-INDUCED HK2 CELLS AND HYPERURICEMIC PATIENTS

Wei-Ting Tseng, Kuan-Da Lee, Ming-Hui Chen, and William T H Chang

Lytone Enterprise, Inc. New Taipei City, 221, Taiwan

Keywords: dipeptide, uric acid, hyperuricemia, HK2 cell

Background: Uric acid (UA) is the end product of purine degradation and a high level of UA may induce gout with symptoms such as muscle spasm, inflammation, joint pains, and muscle fatigue. Many commercialized drugs have been used to treat gout by inhibiting the formation of UA, accelerating the excretion of UA from body, and inhibiting the activity of xanthine oxidase for the conversion xanthine to UA. However, these uricosuric agents simultaneously exhibit a number of side effects. Thus, there is still need for a new drug or a dietary supplement for reducing the level of UA and moderating gout-related symptoms. Dipeptide, carnosine and anserine have been shown to have the activities of increasing the speed of cell mitosis through stimulation of neutrophils, thus potentially strengthening the repairing mechanism of muscle tissues under stress.

Objective: To understand the anti-hyperuricemia effects of anserine dipeptide from fish extract, we investigated the effects of anserine dipeptide on UA levels in fructose-induced HK2 cells and hyperuricemic patients.

Methods: The xanthine oxidase inhibitory activity was assayed spectrophotometrically at 295 nm. The proximal tubular cell line from normal kidney, HK2 cells, were incubated with Keratinocyte-

SFM medium and exposed with fructose in the present of various concentrations of dipeptide. Further, we examined the relation between dipeptide intake and serum UA levels in hyperuricemic adult men. We measured the UA synthesis from the HK2 cells and serum concentrations of UA by Amplex® red uric acid/uricase kit.

Results: *In vitro*, dipeptide (1 and 3 mg/mL) significantly inhibited the activity of xanthine oxidase compared with the non-treatment group by approximately 8 and 27 %. Moreover, 1 and 5 mg/mL dipepitide significantly decreased the UA synthesis from fructose-induced HK2 cells by 10.40 and 12.03 nM. *In vivo*, administration of 1 g dipeptide decreased the serum UA levels after 1 h treatment in hyperuricemic adult men (n=9) by approximately 14%. In addition, subjects (n=31) supplemented with 50 mg/day of dipeptide for 2 weeks significantly reduced the serum UA levels compared with placebo group by approximately 6.78 mg/dl.

Conclusion: Our study demonstrated that anserine dipeptide could decrease the UA levels of hyperuricemic models *in vitro* and *in vivo*. The effects for the anserine dipeptide to treat or protect from hyperuricemia might be related to the xanthine oxidase inhibitory action. We anticipate that the anserine dipeptide derived from fish extracts might serve as a functional food for the prevention or treatment of hyperuricemic patients.

BACTERIAL DIVERSITY AND TECHNOLOGICAL, FUNCTIONAL AND SAFETY CHARACTERIZATION OF NON-STARTER LACTIC ACID BACTERIA STRAINS IN GOAT CHEESES

Zhaoxu Meng, Lanwei Zhang, Xue Han, Huaxi Yi

School of Chemistry and Chemical Engineering, Harbin Institute of Technology, Harbin, 150090, China

Keywords: Bacterial diversity, Non-starter lactic acid bacteria, Technological properties, Functional properties, Safety

Background: Researches on the specific environment of lactic acid bacteria community diversity play an important role in the excavation and utilization of lactic acid bacteria. During the production of goat cheese, people adhere to the fixed starter culture and the optimal fermentation agents are suitable for production of goat cheese have not been studied systematically. Non-starter lactic acid bacteria (NSLAB) dominate cheese microbiota during ripening. They tolerate the hostile environment well, strongly influence the biochemistry of curd maturation, and finally contribute to the development of the characteristics of cheese. NSLAB inhabiting fermented food have been recently improved as probiotic strains. Several NSLAB are selected on the basis of their health benefits and employed in cheese-making. Our study focuses on their application as adjunct cultures, in order to accelerate the cheese ripening process and improve the probiotic function.

Objective: The aim of this work was to study the bacterial diversity of 8 cheese samples made of raw goat milk without thermal treatment and industrial starter, and to perform a first screening for potential technological and functional properties.

Methods: The bacterial diversity of eight nature goat cheese samples collected from France, America, and Brazil were detected by Illumina MiSeq method. In order to select strains for NSLAB to accelerate cheese ripening, Non-starter lactic acid bacteria (NSLAB) strains have been isolated and evaluated for the technological characteristics related to the cheese production such as optimum growth temperature, acidification activity, proteolytic activity, autolytic activity and aminopeptidase activity. Finally, their functional and safety properties and survival rate under gut-related conditions were also studied.

Results: The results showed that 8 cheese samples contained 432 genus, including lactic acid bacteria (*Lactobacillus*), acetic acid bacteria (*Acetobacter*) and *Lactococcus lactis* (*Lactococcus*). With the number of sequence increasing, the OTU tendency number of per samples decreased and finally reached saturation. The composition analysis indicated that the main bacteria of 8 samples was *Lactobacillus*. Further studies showed that all the isolates presented low acidification rate, and the pH did not reach 5.3 after fermented in skimmed milk at 37 °C for 6 h. Among the isolates, acidification ability at 24 h was different from isolate to isolate. The results also displayed that proteolytic activity of lactobacilli strains was between 17.72 and 48.47 mg Gly/L, and FL5 showed the highest value of 48.47 mg Gly/L. The rate of autolysis of the isolates was between 7.45% and 4.77%. FL9 and FL11 showed the maximal autolytic rate of 44.77% and 43.55%, respectively. Through the determination of the aminopeptidase activity of all the isolates using L-leu-pNA as the substrate, FL18, FL33 and FL29 exhibited higher aminopeptidase activity with the value of 71.02, 68.63 and 68.46 U/mg, respectively. In the further studies, FL5 and FL33 were identified as *Lactobacillus rhamnosus* and FL11 was *Lactobacillus paracasei*. FL11 and FL33 had the higher adherent capability to Caco-2 cells (adherence percentages of 36 and 7% respectively).

The inhibitory effects of these probiotic bacteria were evaluated against *Listeria monocytogenes* and *Staphylococcus aureus* in the goat cheese during refrigerated storage. FL33 presented inhibition rate of 7.93% and 24.57% against *S. aureus* on the 14th and 21st day of storage at 10 °C, respectively; against *L. monocytogenes* these values were 12.96 and 32.99%. Positive inhibition rates of FL11 toward *S. aureus* were evaluated on the 1st, 14th and 21st days of storage (16.36%, 11.01% and 3.49%, respectively); and against *L. monocytogenes* only on the 1st day of storage (3.19%).

Conclusion: We conclude that raw goat milk cheese is a potential source of biotechnologically relevant lactobacilli and the *L.rhamnosus* showed better biotechnological properties than *L.paracasei*. It could be deduced that *L.rhamnosus* exhibited an excellent functional and inhibitory properties and the ability of survival in gut-related conditions, which can be further developed for biotechnological applications

FL33 could accelerate the cheese ripening, and improve the texture and flavour. Therefore strains FL33 exhibited potential application value in cheese production. In this study, it was also found that strain FL33 stood out in inhibiting the growth of *S. aureus* and *L.monocytogenes* in goat cheese over refrigerated storage.

GENERATING HIGH FIBRE AND HIGH RESISTANT STARCH BARLEY GRAIN FOR IMPROVING HEALTH INDICES FOR DIABETES AND BOWEL HEALTH

Zhongyi Li, Hong Wang, Min Huang, Chris Konik-Rose

CSIRO Agriculture, Clunies Ross Street, Black Mountain, ACTON, Canberra, ACT 2601, Australia

Keywords: barley, resistant starch, beta-glucan, amylose, fructan, glycaemic index, bowel cancer

Background: Chronic disorder diseases have become widespread health issues in Australia and other countries internationally. In Australia, 18% of the population has cardiovascular disease, 8% have Type II diabetes, 47% of women and 64% of men are overweight and 4,400 deaths per year result from colorectal cancer. These four types of chronic disorder diseases cost Australia more than US$6 billion annually. In the world, there were 420 million people suffering from Type II diabetes in 2015. Nearly 1.4 million new cases of colorectal cancer were diagnosed in 2012, which may possibly reach 2.4 million annually by 2035. The global cost of diabetes is now $825 billion per year. The global cost for new cases of colorectal cancer is estimated to be US$31.6 billion in 2010 and US$47.1 billion by 2030. Consumption of whole grain cereals has been proposed to be an effective approach for reducing the risks of those chronic disorder diseases due to their high fibre and resistant starch contents.

Objective: To generate high fibre and high resistant starch barley grain for improving health indices for chronic diseases.

Methods: Barley cv Himalaya was mutagenized with sodium azide. Grain was analysed for starch, protein, lipid and fibre contents. Breakfast cereals, bread, and muffins were produced from high amylose barley selections. Animal trials were conducted for measuring glycaemic index (GI) and short chain fatty acid

(SCFA) content and pH in the large bowel and stool (Dr. Tony Bird, CSIRO Human Nutrition). The high amylose barley mutation was combined with the amo1 mutant (high amylose glacier) to improve resistant starch (RS) content and yield of barley grain.

Results: A high amylose barley mutant, Himalaya 292 was first identified from the barley grain with modified grain morphology, subsequently shown to be due to loss of function of starch synthase IIa (SSIIa). Grain composition analyses showed that Himalaya 292 contains low starch content at ~30% of grain weight, high amylose content at ~70% of total starch, high beta-glucan content at ~10%, high fructan content at ~11% and high total fibre at ~25%. Animal and human trials showed that the Himalaya 292 grain significantly reduced GI, increased SCFA and reduced pH value.

Conclusion: Our group is studying the relationship between starch structure and nutritional properties of cereal starches. The endosperm of barley grain typically contains ~50-60% starch composed of ~25% amylose and ~75% amylopectin. Starch synthases transfer glucose from ADP-glucose to the non-reducing end of pre-existing α-(1-4)-linked glucosyl chains of starch. Loss of function mutations of starch synthase genes provides a powerful approach to study the roles of starch synthases in the determination of starch structure and grain composition in barley. Some of these changes in starch also make the modified starch less digestible by increasing the level of resistant starch content of barley grains. The loss of function of starch synthase IIa also leads to an increase of grain total fibre content. The functions of this novel high fibre and high RS barley grain in improving the human health will be discussed.

THE PSYCHROTROPHIC BACTERIA DIVERSITY FROM RAW MILK OF NORTH CHINA AND THEIR PROTEOLYTIC PROPERTY

Liang Xin, Lanwei Zhang, Yanhua Cui, Huaxi Yi, Xue Han

School of Chemistry and Chemical Engineering, Harbin Institute of Technology, Harbin, 150000, China

Keywords: psychrotrophic bacteria, diversity, raw milk, proteolytic property

Background: During refrigerated transportation and cold storage of raw milk, psychrotrophic bacteria occupy the dominant place. In addition, most of these bacteria are capable of producing thermoresistant extracellular proteases, which lead to an unacceptable nutritional and organoleptic quality of the final products.

Objective: To understand the negative effect of psychrotrophic bacteria and their protease in refrigerated raw milk, we investigated the diversity and dynamics of raw cow milk bacterial communities during the refrigeration and proteolytic traits of culturable psychrotrophic bacteria in raw cow milk.

Methods: The raw milk samples were collected from the farm bulk tanks of different farms in Beijing (s1), Heihe (s2) and Harbin (s3) of North China. The diversity of milk samples was determined during 3 days of storage at 0~5°C and 5~10°C, respectively. To acquire the V3 region of bacterial 16S rRNA gene, total microbial DNA from the raw milk samples was isolated using the E. Z. N. A. Bacteria DNA Kit (Omega Bio-Tek, Norcross, GA, USA) following the protocol. DGGE was performed at 60°C, employing 8% polyacrylamide gels with a denaturing range of 30-60%.

Electrophoresis was performed at 120 V for 2.16×10^4 s. The band abundance, evenness and Shannon-Wiener index were determined based on the number and relative quantity of the bands. Cluster analysis of the sample profiles was carried out using the unweighted pair group method with arithmetic means (UPGMA). The amplified products of interest in the DGGE profiles were sent for cloning and sequencing. Sequence information was acquired by aligning the results with the sequences in GenBank using the BLAST search program at the National Center for Biotechnology Information (NCBI) (http://www.ncbi.nlm.nih.gov).

Samples for analysis of psychrotrophic bacteria by culturing were incubated at 0~5°C for 10 days. On days 10 of storage, the samples were serially diluted with 0.85% sodium chloride (NaCl) and plated on PCM agar. The plates were incubated at 4°C and observed for up to 10 days. Colonies with different morphologies that grew on PCA plates were picked and subcultured to obtain pure cultures. Proteolytic ability of these isolates was tested using skim milk agar. The presence of clear zones around the colonies was indicative of proteolysis. The identification was confirmed by the 16S rRNA gene sequencing method. The gene sequence was then compared with sequences available in the nucleotide database by using the BLAST algorithm at the NCBI (www.ncbi.nlm.nih.gov). The proteolytic isolates were incubated at 15°C for 72 h. Samples were taken every 24 h, and absorbance at 600 nm was determined. Meanwhile, psychrotrophic bacteria were inoculated in skim milk (pH 6.5) and incubated for up to 72 h at 15°C. Samples were taken every 24 h for the analysis of proteolytic activity.

Results: The dominant bacteria in milk were presumably affiliated with the orders *Pseudomonadales* and *Lactobacillales*. In addition, *Bacillales* was found in every sample, Enterobacteriales was observed in sample B and C. Moreover, Caulobacterales was only identified in sample A, Actinomycetales and Aeromonadales were in sample B, and Flavobacteriales was only in sample C. Significant changes in the bacterial community composition were observed in the samples incubation at 5~10°C. During storage under both conditions, numerous bands affiliated to the order *Pseudomonadales* became visible. The bands that belonged to Enterobacteriales also slightly became brighter during the storage at 0~5°C. By contrast, the intensity of other orders became weak. The dominant bacteria in all the samples were affiliated with the Pseudomonadales after storage. The Shannon-Wiener index of the bacterial community in raw milk samples from sample B was higher than that from other areas. The dendrogram obtained by the cluster analysis for the farm milk samples showed two distinct groups. Samples collected from the same area formed one group.

Meanwhile, 26 psychrotrophic isolates selected as potential protease producer were further identified as *Pseudomonas* by 16S rRNA gene sequencing. According to the ability of producing protease, these isolates were selected for growth and proteolytic activity evaluation at refrigeration temperature 15°C for 72 h. As the storage time elapsed, an increase in number of psychrotrophic bacteria was detected. Highest cell density was observed at the end of 72 h. The isolates 4, 7, 11, 29, 36, 37, 38 and 41 had a considerably higher growth compared to other isolates after 3 days incubation. Max absorbance at 600 nm was observed at 72 h of isolate 29 (0.703 ± 0.002). Meanwhile, the time course of proteolytic activity was followed at 15°C. The proteolytic activity was observed after 24 h incubation, and the proteolysis obtained after 72 h of growth in the skim milk was the highest. Isolate 38 exhibited the highest proteolytic activity with the activity of 5.741 ± 0.003 L-Leu mmol/L.

Conclusion: The composition of psychrotrophic bacterial flora in raw milk play an important role in the determination of milk quality. Monitoring the dominant psychrotrophic species responsible for the production of proteolytic enzymes offers a sensitive and efficient tool for maintaining better milk quality in the milk industry.

PHYTOCHEMICAL AND BIOACTIVE PROPERTIES OF GINGER-FLAVOURED COMPOSITE BISCUIT FROM COMPOSITE FLOUR OF WHEAT, BAMBARA GROUNDNUT AND PLANTAIN

M.O. Oluwamukomi and T.J. Arogundade

Dept of Food Science and Technology, Federal University of Technology, Akure, Nigeria

Keywords: phytochemical, bioactive properties, bambara, plantain, ginger, composite biscuit

Background: Phytochemicals are non-nutritive, bioactive plant compounds in fruits, vegetables, grains and other plant foods that have been linked to reducing the risk of major degenerative diseases. Many phytochemicals have antioxidant activity and reduce the risk of many diseases. Ginger has been consumed worldwide as a spice and flavouring agent from the ancient time. It has some tremendous beneficial effect to human body to cure various types of diseases The production of bread and biscuits from refined wheat flour exclusively has been observed to be deficient in bioactive phytochemicals such as tocopherols and phenolic acids. Inclusion of ginger as a flavour in such products will therefore be of high health benefit.

Objective: The objective of this study was therefore to produce a ginger-flavoured biscuit from flour blends (wheat, Bambara groundnut and plantain flours) at varied proportions with the aim of determining the phytochemical bioactive properties of the food product.

Methods: Composite flour was prepared by blending wheat, bambara groundnut, and plantain flour and the various proportion obtained were flavoured with 2.5% ginger while 100 % wheat flour was used as the control. Biscuits were prepared from the blends. Phytochemical screening of the flour blends was done to detect the presence of alkaloids, flavonoids, saponins and tannins. The flavonoid content was determined using the gravimetric method. The saponin content of the sample was determined by double extraction gravimetric method. Tannin content was determined using photometric while the *alkaloid* was determined by the alkaline precipitation gravimetric method.

Results: Qualitative phytochemical screening revealed that tannin, alkaloid, flavonoid and saponin were present in the flour blends. Tannins concentration ranged between 1.17 to 1.24 mg/100g. The saponin content also ranged between 0.89 and 1.03 mg/100g with biscuit with 68.15% (wheat flour); 17.04% (Bambara groundnut flour); 14.81% (plantain flour);having the lowest value while flour from biscuit with low bambara but higher plantain flour had the highest. The alkaloid concentration in the flour blends ranged between 1.27 and 1.38 mg/100g. In the case of flavonoid, it ranged between 1.23 and 1.33 mg/100g. Total phenolic content ranged from 2.86 to 4.48 mg GAE/g. The total flavonoid content also ranged from 1.65 to 2.87 mg QEAC/g. Total phenol and total flavonoid contents of biscuits with ginger was higher than that of the control (biscuits produced from 100 % wheat flour). This suggests that much of the phenolic compounds might have originated from the incorporation of ginger.

Conclusion: The findings in this study has shown that biscuit containing a combination of ginger powder, Bambara groundnut and unripe plantain flour will be of high potential health benefits and serve as a functional food for prevention of noncommunicable diseases.

INTERACTIONS OF FOOD AND BEVERAGES WITH COMMONLY USED PRESCRIPTION MEDICATIONS

Sheila M. Wicks[a], Garvin Kane, Temitope O. Lawal[b,c], Gail B. Mahady[b]

[a]Department of Clinical Anatomy and Cell Biology, Rush University, Chicago, IL, USA; [b]Division of Cardiovascular Disease & Internal Medicine , Mayo Clinic Rochester MN, USA [c]Department of Pharmacy Practice, University of Illinois at Chicago, Chicago, IL, USA; [d]Department of Pharmaceutical Microbiology, University of Ibadan, Ibadan, Nigeria

Keywords: Drug metabolism; tyramine; CYP3A4; cranberry, grapefruit; HMG-CoA reductase inhibitor; alcohol; caffeine, garlic, ginger

Background: When it comes to prescription medications, patients rarely ask about which foods should be avoided. In some instances, patients should take their medication with a particular food or beverage to aid palatability (and hence compliance), minimize local irritation to the gastrointestinal tract, or aid in drug absorption. However, more importantly, there are many incidences when the consumption of specific foods in combination with certain medications presents a problem by interfering with the absorption, metabolism, or excretion of these drugs. If these instances go unrecognized, there may be significant divergence of therapeutic drug levels, and hence therapeutic effects and possible drug-related adverse events. For example, vitamin K containing foods reduce the efficacy of warfarin, while ginger and garlic have anticoagulant effects and enhance the effects of warfarin.

Objectives: This work will highlight some of the most recent research indicating where concomitant ingestion of particular foods or beverages can interfere with prescription drug safety and efficacy and then reviews how a better understanding of these interactions can sometimes be used to aid in patient management.

Methods: We look at examples of food-drug interactions:

Effects of Vitamin K on Warfarin Anticoagulation

The anticoagulant effect of warfarin is mediated through inhibition of the vitamin K-dependent coagulation factors II, VII, IX, and X. A key feature in the stability of the warfarin anticoagulant effect is week-to-week differences in the content of vitamin K in the diet. Foods particularly high in vitamin K include vegetable oils, asparagus, broccoli, Brussels sprouts, cabbage, lettuce, parsley, peas, pickles, and spinach. Many dietary supplements, including multivitamin preparations and herbal products, are also high in vitamin K, which can affect coagulation.

Monoamine Oxidase Inhibitors and Tyramine

Monoamine oxidase (MAO) inhibitors, used in the treatment of depression and phobic anxiety disorders, are being increasingly replaced by safer alternatives due to a number of potentially dangerous interactions with foods containing high levels of tyramine (e.g., beer, ale, red wine, soy, aged cheeses, smoked or pickled fish or meat, anchovies, yeast, and vitamin supplements). Ingested tyramine is normally metabolized by the enzyme MAO in the bowel wall and liver.

Calcium Impairs Absorption of certain Antibiotics

Calcium-rich foods, such as dairy products and tofu, even milk added to tea or coffee, are sufficient to significantly impede the absorption of several antibiotics, including tetracycline, minocycline, doxycycline, levofloxacin, and ciprofloxacin

Ginger Enhances Anticoagulant Effects

Ginger is a widely used condiment, food, and herbal medicine. It is used as a digestive aid, to treat inflammation, for morning sickness, but also has antiplatelet and antimicrobial effects. Ginger therefore has the potential to interact with anticoagulants. In the scientific literature, there are a few reports of an increase in the International Normalized Ratio (INR) in patients taking ginger root, ginger tea, and other herbal medicines containing ginger, in conjunction with warfarin (2). The INR is an alternate measure of the common coagulation test known as prothrombin time (PT), and was introduced by the World Health Organization. A normal INR is approximately 0.9 to 1.1 and is elevated to between 2-3.5 when patients are on warfarin therapy, so an elevation in the case of ginger supplementation indicates that ginger has anticoagulant effects.

Garlic Enhances Anticoagulant Effects and Reduces Protease Inhibitor Levels

Garlic (known scientifically as Allium sativum L.) is both a food and a dietary supplement, and its effects are well documented because of its beneficial effects on health (3, 4). Garlic contains phytochemicals that may influence the pharmacokinetic and pharmacodynamic behaviors of prescription drugs. However, the compounds contained in garlic have shown inconsistent effects on the cytochrome P450 isoenzymes. Clinical reports show a possible interaction with garlic (primarily as a dietary supplement) and warfarin. acetaminophen and lisinopril (3,4). In addition, garlic and garlic supplements have a significant impact on the efficacy of protease inhibitors used to treat human immunodeficiency virus (HIV).

Soy Reduces Anticoagulant Effects

Soybeans (Glycine max) are fermented and then used as part of a wide array of Asian cuisine and soy-based products. These fermented products are well known to contain high levels of vitamin K that may interact with anticoagulants. Clinical reports and studies have shown that the administration of warfarin along with soy protein, soymilk, or other soy products may decrease the INR in patients (2).

Results: Specific Examples of Food- Drug Interactions

Table 1. Drug–food Interactions

Drug	Food Interaction	Reference
Acetaminophen	Alcohol ↑ AE	5
Artemether	Grapefruit ↑ DE	6
Atorvastatin	Grapefruit ↑ DE	5, 6
	Alcohol ↑ AE	
Buspirone	Grapefruit ↑ DE	6, 7
Carbamazepine	Grapefruit ↑ DE	5, 6
	Alcohol ↑ AE	
Celecoxib & other NSAIDs	Alcohol ↑AE	5
Cefotetan	Alcohol ↑ AE	5
Cilostazol	Grapefruit ↑ DE	6
Ciprofloxacin	Dairy, Ca, Mg, Fe ↓ DE	1
Clomipramine	Grapefruit ↑ DE	6
Clozapine	Caffeine ↑ DE	5, 8
	Alcohol ↑ AE	
Cyclosporine	Grapefruit ↑ DE	6, 9
Diazepam	Grapefruit ↑ DE	5, 6
	Alcohol ↑ AE	
Doxycycline	Dairy, Ca, Mg, Fe ↓ DE	1
Ebastine	Grapefruit ↑ DE	6
Felodipine	Grapefruit ↑ DE	6, 9
Grisecfulvin	Alcohol ↑ AE	5
Fe supplements	Food ↓ effect	10
Isocarboxazid	Tyramine ↑ AE	10
Isoniazid	Alcohol ↑ AE	5
	Tyramine ↑ AE	
Isosorbide dinitrate	Alcohol ↑ DE	5
Levofloxacin	Dairy, Ca, Mg, Fe ↓ DE	1
Lithium	Caffeine ↓ DE	8
Loratadine	Grapefruit ↑ DE	6, 7
Linezolid	Alcohol, caffeine, tyramine ↑ AE	5, 8
Lovastatin	Grapefruit ↑ DE	6
Methadone	Grapefruit ↑ DE	6

Metronidazole	Alcohol, ↑ AE	5
Midazolam	Grapefruit ↑ DE	6
Minocycline	Dairy, Ca, Mg, Fe ↓ DE	1
Nimodipine	Grapefruit ↑ DE	6, 7
Nisoldipine	Grapefruit ↑ DE	6
Nitrofurantoin	Alcohol ↑ AE	5
Phenelzine	Tyramine ↑ AE	5
Pranidipine	Grapefruit ↑ DE	6
Saquinavir	Grapefruit ↑ DE Garlic [Symbol] DE	3, 4, 6
Sertraline	Grapefruit ↑ DE Alcohol ↑ AE	5, 6
Sildenafil	Grapefruit ↑ DE	6
Simvastatin	Grapefruit ↑ DE	6
Sulfa drugs	Alcohol ↑ AE	5
Tacrolimus	Grapefruit ↑ DE	6
Terfenadine	Grapefruit ↑ DE	6
Tetracycline	Dairy, Ca, Mg, Fe ↓ effect	1
Theophylline	Caffeine ↑ DE	8

Methods:Thyroid hormone	Food ↓ effect	10
Tranylcypromine	Tyramine ↑ AE	10
Triazolam	Grapefruit ↑ DE	6
Warfarin	Vitamin K-rich foods ↓ DE Garlic [Symbol] DE Cranberry [Symbol] DE Green tea [Symbol] DE Soy [Symbol] DE Ginger [Symbol] DE	2, 3, 11, 12
Zaleplon	Grapefruit ↑ DE	6
Zolpidem	Alcohol ↑AE	5

[a]This list is not meant to be exhaustive but merely highlighting some of the main food and beverages that may give rise to a clinically significant interaction with particular drugs. Ca, calcium; Mg, magnesium; Fe, iron; AE, adverse effects; DE, drug effects

Conclusions: We have reviewed some of the most common drug interactions with food and beverages. By acting on gastric motility, pH, and drug metabolism, food and beverages can have a variety of effects on the absorption and metabolism of medications, as well as on many vitamins and minerals, with the clinical significance ranging from passing interest to concern for significant reductions in drug action, as is seen with garlic and saquinavir, as well as serious adverse events, as seen with cranberry and warfarin. For some food-drug interactions, such as grapefruit juice, that affect drug metabolism through the cytochrome P450 isoenzymes, there is huge variability from one person to the next and the risks of dangerous interactions are only present in a few. With further understanding and perhaps profiling of patients for their gene expression of metabolic enzymes, it may be possible to identify those most at risk for both beverage-drug and drug-drug interactions. In the meantime, it is best for patients to take their medications with a glass of water unless otherwise advised.

References:

1. Jung H, Peregrina AA, Rodriguez JM, Moreno-Esparza R. The influence of coffee with milk and tea with milk on the bioavailability of tetracycline. Biopharm Drug Dispos 1997;18:459–63.
2. Ge B, Zhang Z, Zuo Z. Updates on the clinical evidenced herb-warfarin interactions. Evid Based Complement Alternat Med. 2014;2014:957362.
3. Berginc K, Kristl A. The mechanisms responsible for garlic, drug interactions and their in vivo relevance. Current Drug Metabolism 2013;14:90-101.
4. Piscitelli SC1, Burstein AH, Welden N, Gallicano KD, Falloon J. The effect of garlic supplements on the pharmacokinetics of saquinavir. Clin Infect Dis. 2002;34:234-8.
5. Fraser AG. Pharmacokinetic interactions between alcohol and other drugs. Clin Pharmacokinet 1997;33:79–90.

6. Kane GC, Lipsky JJ. Drug-grapefruit juice interactions. Mayo Clin Proc 2000;5:933–42

TRACED TUSCAN FOOD FOR BREAST-CANCER SURGERY-TREATED PATIENTS UNDER CHEMOTHERAPY: A PROGRAM FOR A CLINICAL TRIAL AT THE BREAST CENTER OF PISA-ITALY UNIVERSITY HOSPITAL

Enrica Bargiacchi[1], Annalisa Romani[2], Patrizia Pinelli[2], Manuela Roncella[3], Andrea Michelotti[4], Ilaria Montagnani[1], Sergio Miele[1]

[1]Consortium INSTM, Via G. Giusti 9, 50121 Firenze, Italy; [2]Phytolab-DiSIA Univ. Firenze (Italy); [3]Breast Center, Dep. of Breast Surgery, Pisa Univ. Hospital, Pisa, Italy; [4]O.U. Medical Oncology I, Pisa Univ. Hospital, Pisa, Italy

Keywords: Fortified foods, antioxidants, polyphenols, chemotherapy

Background: Patients' stress after discovering to be affected by breast cancer, the related surgery treatment, and the effects of pharma, chemotherapy and radiotherapy are conditions leading to increased oxidative stress. Previous research indicated that diets based on food and supplements high in natural antioxidants help to control the free radicals and oxidative stress-related blood parameters, with increased patients' wellness. We have studied Tuscany food ingredients, founding that in several cases they have an edge in terms of polyphenols and other bioactive molecule contents. Starting from the excellence of Tuscany traced food, We prepared a new set of foods, herbal teas, and supplements to be clinically tested in the project TUSCANY NATURBEN.

Objective: To carry out a clinical trial aiming at evaluating chemo-induced toxicity during the adjuvant chemotherapy in radically surgery-treated patients for breast carcinoma, both in a control group (free diet) and a test group (diet including +3 free daily choices of fortified foods). Also blood free radicals, and

287

antioxidant capacity are monitored, and pleasantness of food is evaluated.

Methods: Tuscan traced foods, herbal teas, and supplements, sensorially appealing for taste, aroma, and "roundness", were prepared, analytically characterized for their dietary, antioxidant and anti-radical constituents (analyses presented). The clinical trial protocol will consider diet administration in the period between 2nd-5th chemotherapy cycles at the Breast Center of the University Hospital of Pisa-Tuscany (Italy). Psycho-physical wellness, and oxidative stress-related blood parameters (tested by CR-4000 of Callegari-Italy) of the control and treated groups of patients will be controlled through and after the test period. The treated group also will express their evalutation on the administered foods.

Results: So far, only data on the analytical characterization and sensorial evaluation of the foods, herbal teas, and supplements are available, as the clinical trial is still in progress. However, we have already achieved some important preliminary results: (i) it is the first time that a multi-disciplinary team, from biotechnologists to MD, work together to tune up a diet to reduce drawbacks of after-breast surgery chemotherapy in patients; (ii) we set a guideline for presenting a request of authorization of a clinical trial concerning alternative food and diets to an Italian Ethical Committee; (iii) we had foods, herbal teas, and supplements with consistent nutraceutical characteristics available at distribution level and positively evaluated by group of patients; (iv) we preliminary tested the responsiveness of the equipment used to check the oxidative stress-related blood parameters.

Conclusion: This clinical trial has been intended by this multi-disciplinary research team as a preliminary tuning activity for a larger experiment, aiming at improving patients' wellness during chemotherapy.

Acknowledgement: Regione Toscana (Italy) for funding TUSCANY-NATURBEN Project (D.D. 2014/4361).

THE BENEFICIAL EFFECTS OF BERRY FRUIT ON COGNITIVE AND NEURONAL FUNCTION IN AGING

Barbara Shukitt-Hale[1], Marshall G. Miller[1], Nopporn Thangthaeng[1], Derek R. Fisher[1], Donna F. Bielinski[1], Megan E. Kelly[1], and Tammy Scott[1]

[1]Neuroscience and Aging Lab., USDA-ARS Human Nutrition Research Center on Aging at Tufts University, Boston, MA 02111

Keywords: berries, cognition, aging

Research has demonstrated, in both human and animals, that cognition decreases with age, to include deficits in processing speed, executive function, memory, and spatial learning. The cause of these functional declines is not entirely understood; however, neuronal losses and the associated changes in the activity of neurotransmitters, secondary messengers, and their receptors may be caused by long term increases in and susceptibility to oxidative stress and inflammation. Therefore, one approach to improving neuronal functioning might be to alter the neuronal environment to reduce the impact of oxidative and inflammatory stressors. Research conducted in our laboratory, initially with animals but more recently with humans, has shown that consumption of berry fruits, i.e., strawberries and blueberries, which are high in polyphenolics, can prevent and even reverse age-related cognitive and neuronal deficits. The polyphenolic compounds found in these foods may exert their beneficial effects indirectly, through their ability to lower oxidative stress and inflammation, or directly, by altering neuronal structure and signaling involved in neuronal communication. Additionally, the polyphenolics in different berry fruits may have differential effects on cognition and inflammation/oxidative stress. Therefore, dietary interventions with polyphenolic-rich foods may be one strategy to forestall or even reverse age-related neuronal deficits.

LONG CHAIN OMEGA-3 FATTY ACIDS, COGNITIVE AGING, AND DEMENTIA

T.M. Scott

[1]Jean Mayer USDA Human Nutrition Research Center on Aging at Tufts University, Boston, MA, USA

Keywords: omega-3 fatty acids, cognition, aging, dementia

It is estimated that 13.5 million Americans will suffer effects of dementia by the year 2050. These projections have far reaching implications for Medicare, informal care, and long-term institutional care costs. Identifying strategies that may contribute to even minor delays in the progression of cognitive impairment, or onset of diagnosable dementia, would significantly improve the projected impact of these conditions. One promising cost-effective approach to mitigating risk of impairment, or decline, of cognition is dietary modification. The very long-chain omega-3 fatty acids, eicosapentaenoic acid (EPA) and docosahexaenoic acid (DHA), have shown cognitive benefit in aging populations, and are hypothesized to protect brain health via their numerous structural and functional roles in the central nervous system, secondarily via a reduced risk of cardiovascular disease and stroke, and through modulation of the inflammatory response. EPA and DHA are obtained in the diet predominantly from fatty fish, but the diets of many Americans fall short of the 2010 U.S. Dietary Guidelines recommendation, based on cardiovascular benefits, of 8 or more ounces of seafood per week. Data from the Nutrition and Memory in the Elderly and Boston Puerto Rican Health Studies cohorts suggested that individuals whose intake of EPA+DHA at least met the dietary guidelines were over two times less likely to experience cognitive decline over two years, and that higher EPA+DHA intake and DHA concentrations in plasma were associated with greater total brain volume and less cortical atrophy on MRI. Our findings are consistent with experimental evidence and suggest a neuroprotective role for EPA and DHA in the aging human brain. Efforts to increase dietary long chain omega-3 fatty acid intake may provide benefit for quality of life and continued independence of adults as they age.

LINKAGE OF DIET AND INFLAMMATION: MEASURING C-REACTIVE PROTEIN IN EXPERIMENTAL MICE GIVEN VARIABLE DIETS

Gaby Fahmy[1], Erin Lynch[2] and Anju Mathews[3]

Department of Natural Sciences, School of Arts and Science, Felician University, New Jersey, U.S.A

Keywords: c-reactive protein, inflammation, obesity, atherosclerosis, diet,

Background: C-reactive protein (CRP) is an important marker of the inflammatory process, it is produced by the liver in response to inflammation and is considered one of the acute phase proteins. A rise in this protein is an indication of a risk to developing atherosclerosis and coronary artery diseases which might lead to heart attacks. There are many injurious agents that lead to inflammation such as physical, chemical and infectious agents. Certain food types have been also linked to inflammation, while others are considered to be anti-inflammatory.

Objective: To evaluate the effect of different diets on the levels of c-reactive protein in the plasma of experimental animals as an indication of inflammation.

Methods: 11 mice were divided into 4 groups, including a control group and 3 other groups, which were given each a different diet. Two mice were given a regular mouse diet, 3 mice were fed a high fat diet, 3 mice were fed a red meat diet, and 3 mice were fed a diary diet. The exposure of these diets lasted 7 weeks. Over the course of the experiment, the mice were placed on their appropriate diets in the same environment and were closely observed. At the end of the time interval, blood plasma samples will be taken to measure the C-reactive protein by ELISA immunoassay.

Results: Control mice had the following levels of absorbance 1.329 & 3.174. Meat fed mice had the following values: 1.054, 0.329 & 0.352. Cheese (dairy) fed mice had the following values:

0.252, 0.316 & 0.080. High sugar fed mice showed the following levels: 0.629 & 0.290. As it can be seen, the two mice within the control group had the highest CRP levels, while one of the mice within the meat group followed close behind. After these three mice, the mice with the next highest CRP level was from the sugar group, with 0.629 absorption. Every other mouse, especially the three mice who were pregnant and gave birth, had very low CRP levels.

Conclusion: Our study demonstrated that the variable diets did not clearly increase the levels of c-reactive protein as a marker of acute inflammation. The mice that were not given the regular mice food had lower levels of C-reactive protein than the control group. Besides the control group, one mouse in the meat group also had high CRP levels, which may lead one to believe that red meat may also cause elevated CRP levels. Presented with these results, it is safe to say that further testing over a longer time interval is required for activation of the production of CRP.

NEWBOULDIA LAEVIS MODULATES B-CELL FUNCTION, IMPROVES INSULIN SENSITIVITY, AND ATTENUATES ATHEROGENIC DYSLIPIDAEMIA IN DIABETIC RATS

Okafor Jane[1,5], Erukainure Ochuko[1], Ajiboye John[2], Etoamaihe Michael[1], Okafor Gabriel[3], and Awoniyi Sunday[4]

[1]Nutrition and Toxicology Division, Federal Institute of Industrial Research, Lagos, Nigeria; [2]College of Natural and Applied Sciences, Bells University of Technology, Ota, Nigeria; [3]Department of Food Science and Technology, University of Nigeria, Enugu State Nigeria; [4]College of Medicine, University of Lagos, Lagos, Nigeria; [5]Food Science and Technology Department, Cape Peninsula University of Technology, Bellville, 7535, South Africa.

Keywords: Atherogenic Indices; β – Cell function; Dyslipidemia; and Insulin Sensitivity

Background: The increasing number of people with diabetes, especially in most developing countries, has become a major global health issue. Diabetes has been described as a metabolic disorder characterized by hyperglycaemia, which affects carbohydrate, protein and lipid metabolism. It may be due to inadequate insulin secretion as seen in type 1 diabetes or insulin resistance seen in type 2 diabetes. Because of the side effects of some synthetic drugs, there has been an increasing interest in complementary and alternative medicine like medicinal plants and herbs in the management of diabetes. *Newbouldia laevis.* (*Bignoniaceae* family) is a medicinal plant popularly used in folk or traditional medicine for the treatment of many diseases, including diabetes. Despite the wide use of this plant in traditional medicine, there is limited scientific evidence/proof to support these claims of therapeutic effects and proof of efficacy.

Objective: To understand the therapeutic potentials/properties of *Newbouldia laevis* in diabetes treatment by investigating the antidiabetic and/or hypoglycaemic effects of the aqueous ethanol extract of *N. laevis* leaves in alloxan–induced diabetic rats.

Methods: Acclimatized rats were divided into seven groups. Diabetes was induced by a single injection of alloxan in all groups except for groups 1, 6 and 7. Group 1 served as the control. Group 2 served as the negative control; group 3 was treated with metformin + glibenclamide; while groups 4 and 5 were treated with extracts of 200 and 400 mg/kg bw respectively; groups 6 and 7 were given only the *Newbouldia* extracts of 200 and 400 mg/kg bw respectively. After 21 days of treatment, the rats were sacrificed by cervical dislocation. Blood serum was analyzed to evaluate insulin levels, β cell function, insulin sensitivity, lipid profile and atherogenic indices.

Results: All treated groups showed significant ($p < 0.05$) reduction in fasting blood glucose level, total cholesterol, triglyceride, LDL and increased HDL levels. An improved serum insulin level, β cell function, and increased insulin sensitivity were also observed in all treated groups except for group 5 which was treated with 400 mg/kg of *N.laevis* extract which had a rather low β – cell function.

Conclusion: Our study demonstrated that aqueous ethanol extract of *N. laevis.* possess potent antidiabetic properties/effects, which was evident from the reduction in fasting blood glucose level, total cholesterol, triglyceride, LDL and increased HDL levels. This may be due to the result or consequence of modulation of the β-cell function and increased insulin sensitivity. Treatment with 200 mg/kg bw of the extract had better conclusive, beneficial effects.

AUTHOR INDEX

Diaz-Cintra S	86	
Dibekçi M	117	
Dillon C	68	
Doghor P	83	
Doğuç DK	158	
Domingo JF	104	
Donohue D	231	
Dwyer JT	107	
Elliott-Theberge K	83	
Emenaker NJ	107	
Emoto N	61	
Erdoğan FS	115	
Erukainure O	295	
Esteghamati A	51	64
Etoamaihe M	295	
Fahmy G	293	
Fernández-Gomez B	248	
Fernando W	166	
Filipek A	182	
Fisher DR	288	
Foor A	83	
Fukuoka J	100	
Furusato B	100	
Geigle PR	75	
Giannone J	234	
Go JRJ	93	
Goco MEC	93	
Gorman PH	75	
Guo C	260	
Guo CH	184	
Guo QQ	184	
Gupta V	83	
Guzmán-Gerónimo RI	215	
Guzmán-Pérez V	58	
Ha JM	219	
Hackl T	237	

Kalala F	83		
Kane G	280		
Karam M	110		
Karaushu O	71		
Kawada H	260		
Kawasaki Y	129		
Khan IN	255	257	
Kelly ME	288		
Kim D	219		
Kim J	134		
Kim J	134		
Kim J	219		
Kindel T	234		
Kiss AK	182		
Kittibunchakul S	198		
Konik-Rose C	272		
Krause D	32		
Kumar P	38	46	217
Kurtulmus S	115		
Labiano DF	93		
Labriaga KM	104		
Larry M	51	64	
LaSpina M	250		
Lastrilla HAS	104		
Lawal TO	280		
Layug RA	93		
Lee DG	219		
Lee KD	267		
Lee KW	134		
Lee S	134		
Lei P	112	127	
Li K	127		
Li W	152		
Li Z	272		
Lin H	225		
Lin K	171		

Lintag EIBS	104	
Liu F	40	
Liu X	112	127
Longvah T	255	
Lorenzetti A	71	
Lu WW	177	
Lynch E	293	
Lyu L	243	
MacDonald A	231	
MacDonald- Wicks L	148	
Mahady GB	280	
Manalastas KNM	104	
Mann MLC	104	
Mantello A	71	
Marcellino M	71	
Marcuard S	234	
Marotta F	71	
Martín MÁ	248	
Martinez-Saez N	239	
Martirosyan D	25	
Mathews A	293	
Mathur S	83	
Matsuo T	100	143
Mattarei A	250	
McEvoy M	148	
Meng Z	269	
Mesa MD	248	
Mewis I	58	
Michelotti A	286	
Miele S	286	
Miller MG	288	
Miranda RFP	104	
Mirmiranpour H	51	64
Mitchell A	25	
Mittal M	38	
Miyata Y	100	143

Mizuno M	175	
Montagnani I	286	
Moodley R	189	192
Mora-Escobedo R	215	
Morales P	246	
Moriya T	129	
Mrvichin N	140	
Mutoh M	102	
Nakamura Y	143	
Nakhjavani M	51	64
Namini NK	179	
Naruszewicz M	182	
Nascimento LCS	122	
Nealon R	136	
Nehmi A	262	
Nguyen TH	219	
Nishihira J	129	
Nishimura M	129	
Nishino H	133	
Nolan R	234	
Noureddine T	262	
Nwanna EE	164	
Oboh G	164	
Ogunlaja OO	189	192
Oh SR	80	
Ohba K	100	143
Okafor G	295	
Okafor J	295	
Oliveri MA	42	
Oluwamukomi MO	278	
On-nom N	186	201
Ozdemir O	265	
Pala R	265	
Palma XE	42	
Paradisi C	250	
Parde DKS	93	

Patterson A	148		
Penna ALB	122	124	
Perez-Cruz C	86	215	
Pérez-Grijalva B	215		
Pereze AGA	93		
Perricone NV	140		
Persson N	54		
Pfeiffer AFH	58		
Pinelli P	286		
Plakida A	90		
Polański JA	182		
Possonato-Vieira JS	96		
Pourpak Z	179		
Prasad AS	210		
Preuss HG	38	46	140
Preuss HG	217		
Preuss JM	140		
Randazzo J	260		
Renteria J	83		
Riley M	32		
Riscuta G	126		
Risinger C	54		
Rodriguez IJY	93		
Rodriguez LM	107		
Romani A	286		
Roncella M	286		
Rupasinghe HPV	166		
Sabetkish N	179		
Sagara Y	100		
Sahasakul Y	186		
Sahin K	265		
Sahin N	265		
Saito N	61		
Sakaguchi K	175		
Sakai F	129		
Sakai H	100	143	

Sánchez KV	239		
Sandrim VC	96		
Santos III AF	93		
Sapwarobol S	186	198	
Savaş MC	158		
Schmidt FL	228		
Schreiner M	58		
Schwedhelm E	237		
Scott T	288	291	
Scott WH	75		
Sergio NL	93		
Seydim AC	117	158	204
Seydim ZBG	115	117	158
Seydim ZBG	204		
Shaheen N	255	257	
Shan Y	112	127	195
Sharma S	83		
Shi YG	184		
Shirai Y	48	61	175
Shoormasti RS	179		
Shukitt-Hale B	288		
Si JB	219		
Silva LF	122	124	
Simbulan RJB	93		
Sincioco JEM	93		
Singh M	192		
Sirjani M	179		
Smith C	152		
Smith JE	75		
Solimene U	71		
Somboonpanyakul P	186	198	
Song YS	80		
Sorkin BC	107		
Srichamnong W	201		
Stefanson AL	208		
Stonehouse W	32		

Suttisansanee U	186	198	201
Swaroop A	38	46	217
Szewczyk J	234		
Tang Q	40		
Taragano FE	68		
Tas TK	115	204	
Tayebi B	179		
Thangthaeng N	288		
Thiyajai P	201		
Tian S	195		
Tiangco MAP	93		
Tipoe GL	177		
Tomono S	102		
Torralba CMC	104		
Torres NTY	86		
Trumbo P	24		
Tseng WT	267		
Tukun AB	255	257	
Tungsuphoom N	186		
Tuzcu M	265		
Ueda S	48	61	
Usenko E	90		
Valenciano AC	104		
Vargas ALP	86		
Vega RC	239		
Verma N	38		
Vicente JCD	104		
Villano KB	104		
Wakabayashi K	102		
Wang H	222		
Wang H	272		
Wang X	80		
Wegener CB	161		
Welinder C	54		
Wendel U	54		
Westendorf J	237		

Whelan J	231		
Wick SM	280		
Wong R	136		
Wright C	83		
Xia Z	177		
Xin L	274		
Xue C	40		
Yagi K	61		
Yamanoue M	48	61	
Yasuda T	143		
Yi H	169	171	269
Yi H	274		
Yotpinta N	186		
Yu M	253		
Yu Z	80		
Zhang J	169	274	
Zhang L	169	171	243
Zhang L	269		
Zhang L	177		
Zhang N	184		
Zhang Z	152		
Zhao Y	231		
Zhou D	225		
Zhuravl'ova T	90		
Zoratti M	250		

Functional and Medical Foods for Chronic Diseases: Bioactive Compounds and Biomarkers

Edited by Danik Martirosyan, PhD and Bruce Burnett, PhD

Editorial Assistant: April Mitchell and Rebecca McCarthy

Made in the USA
Middletown, DE
04 September 2016